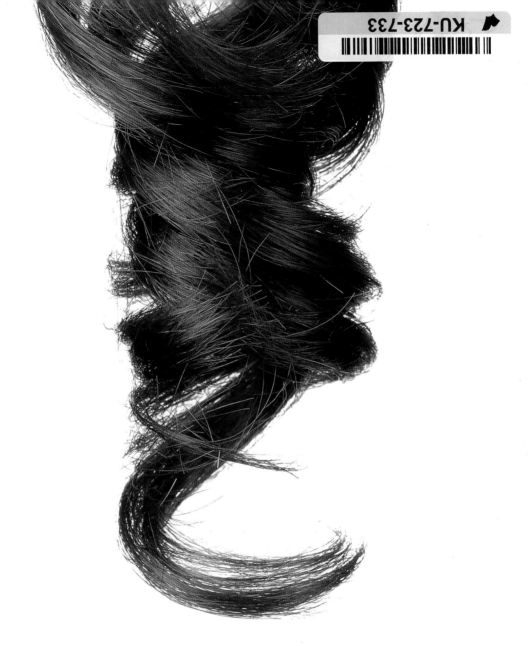

city hair

THIS IS A CARLTON BOOK

Text (except pages 10, 30, 54 and 78), design, illustrations
and photography copyright © 2000 Carlton Books Limited
Text pages 10, 30, 54 and 78 copyright © 2000 Karen Wheeler
Original idea and concept copyright © 2000 Charles Worthington Ltd

This edition was published by Carlton Books Limited in 2000
20 Mortimer Street
London W1T 3JW

A CIP catalogue record for this book is available from the British Library

ISBN paperback 1 84222 134 5
ISBN hardback 1 84222 218 X

The author, licensor and publisher have made every effort to ensure that all information is correct and
up to date at the time of publication. Neither the author, licensor or publisher can accept responsibility
for any accident, injury or damage that results from using the ideas, information or advice offered.

The application and quality of hair products and treatments, herbal preparations and essential oils is beyond
the control of the above parties, who cannot be held responsible for any problems resulting from their use.
Always follow the manufacturer's instructions and if in doubt, seek further advice.

Do not use herbal preparations or essential oils without prior consultation with a qualified practitioner or
medical doctor if you are pregnant, taking any form of medication, or if you suffer from oversensitive skin.
Half-doses of essential oils should always be used for children and the elderly.

No resemblance is intended to any person, living or dead, in the fiction element of this book.
The events and the characters who take part in them have no relation to actual events or living people.

Text: Carmel Allen
Fiction text pages 10, 30, 54 and 78: Karen Wheeler
Photographer (model): Hugh Arnold
Photographer (still life): Patrice de Villiers
Illustrator: Jason Brooks
Stylist: Sophie Kenningham
Make-up: Maggie Hunt and Chase Aston
Editorial Manager: Venetia Penfold
Art Director: Penny Stock
Senior Art Editor: Barbara Zuñiga
Project Editor: Zia Mattocks
Designer: Joanne Long
Production Controller: Janette Davis

Printed and bound in Dubai

city hair

Charles Worthington

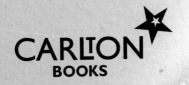

CARLTON
BOOKS

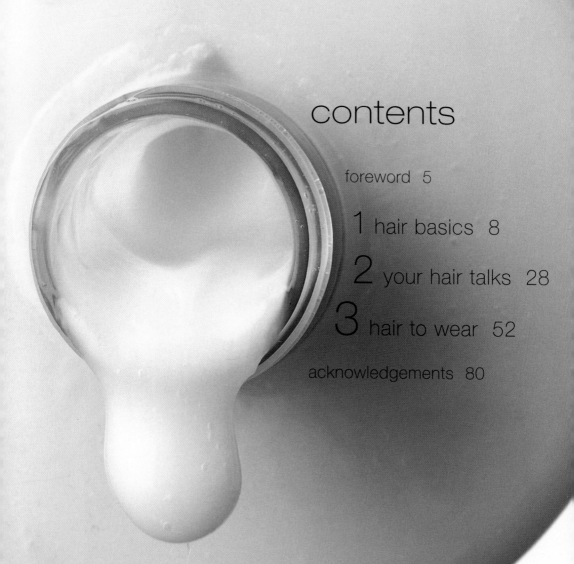

contents

foreword

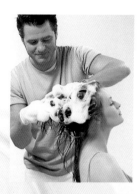

I defy anyone to underestimate the power of hair and its ability to transform the way you look and feel! What's important to me, as a hairdresser who has witnessed and enjoyed the buzz that people get from a great cut or a new style, is to make fabulous hair accessible to everyone. That way, you can enjoy hair that is in peak condition and fulfilling its maximum potential. Most of all, though, I think hair should be fun – it should be about enjoying your individuality and finding a hairstyle that suits you and your lifestyle. *City Hair* aims to make your life easier and answers your everyday hair needs, whether you are having a 'stressed' hair day or get caught out with an amazing invitation for an after-work party with only 20 minutes to transform yourself. I hope that this book helps you to achieve and maintain salon-style hair every day of the week.

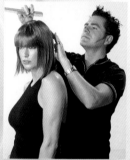

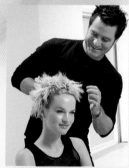

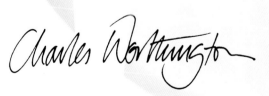

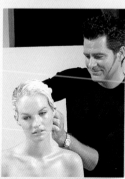

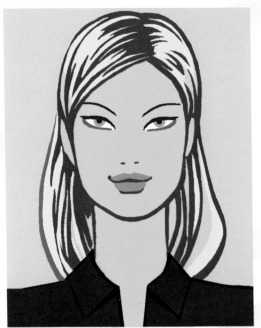

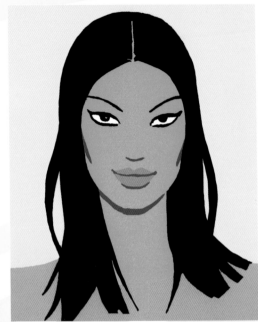

polly

jaz

Polly is a City career babe – traditional, yes, but she's got a twist. Her double first in maths means she can tot up her buying splurges as fast as the computers at Visa. A regular visitor to her Shepherd's Bush home is her boyfriend Harry – a good enough bloke but inclined to be insensitive; money is his aphrodisiac. Even he doesn't know that Polly's sleek blonde hair is the result of painstaking styling to iron out its natural wave. Deep down Polly dreams of a life in the country growing veg, but for now the organic counter at the supermarket has to suffice.

Jaz (short for Jasmine) is your regular club bunnie. She loves all things hip, cool and girlie. Her earliest memory is of dressing up in the contents of her mother's over-stuffed wardrobe – and clothes are still her greatest passion. She can't remember the last time she took off her make-up before going to bed but, with her long, thick, glossy black hair, she always looks stunning nevertheless. She lives to shop – and works in one, too. A stylist in the making, she's often found organizing her shoe collection into boxes labelled with polaroids for easy access.

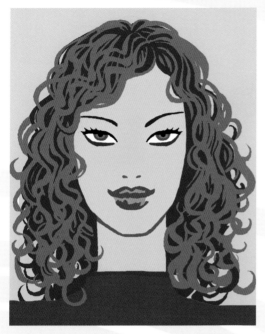

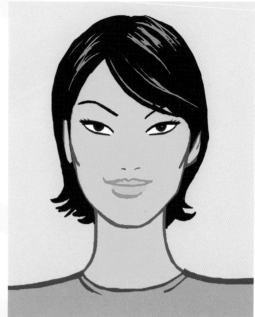

kate

laura

Kate looks like a pre-Raphaelite painting: unruly curly titian hair, milky complexion and rosy cheeks. She works as a personal assistant to the marketing director of Crunch biscuits – not a good career choice when you have a sweet tooth and are prone to overindulgence. Kate is a hopeless romantic who spends many an hour staring out of the window, daydreaming of spending weekends in exotic destinations with her boss on whom she has a hopeless crush. He, on the other hand, is too busy climbing up the career ladder to notice …

Laura is a tomboy: lean and androgynous with a short crop. Her uniform is urban cool – more combats and trainers than pencil skirts and kitten heels. Her only concession to femininity is the occasional understated hair accessory – but nothing pink and definitely not glittery. Laura loves to work out but is fiercely competitive and intimidates most of her fellow gym-goers. She's a TV researcher on a nature series – not quite her cup of tea; she wants to make gritty documentaries and dreams of winning a BAFTA (the acceptance speech is well-rehearsed).

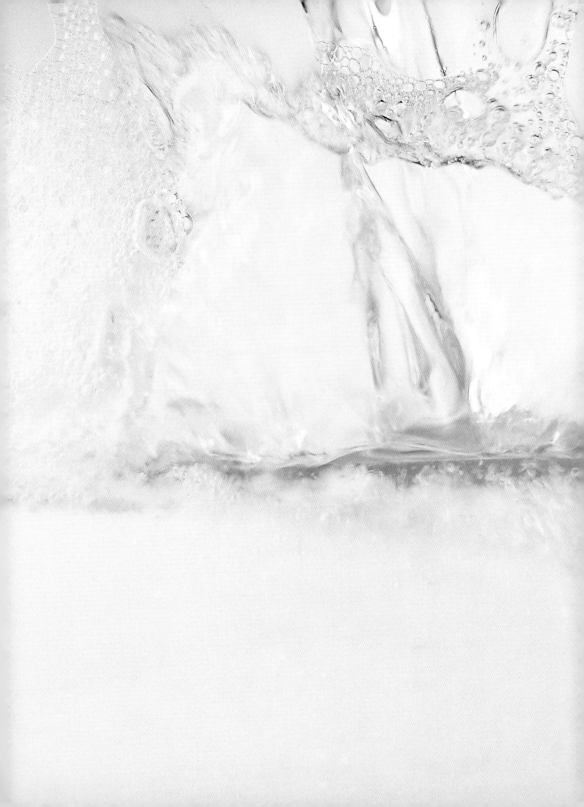

hair basics

home, sweet home

'**Oh, Polly,**' **moaned Kate,** tossing back her unruly red curls and flinging herself down perilously on Polly's new cream sofa, glass of red wine in hand. 'I can't believe you've agreed to let Chrissie come and stay for a month – what a nightmare.' Polly did indeed know that Chrissie could be high-maintenance (to say the least), but then so, too, could Kate. She grimaced as a drop of wine from Kate's glass splashed onto her candy-striped pyjamas, but at least it didn't hit the sofa.

With the help of her parents (rich) and her first city bonus, Perfect Polly – as the others called her in their more green-eyed moments – had bought a four-bedroom house in Shepherd's Bush, chosen largely for its proximity to fashionable, but much more expensive, Notting Hill. Polly had proceeded to install her BFs: Laura, her best friend from Manchester University and her two oldest friends from school in Southampton, fashion-mad Jaz and, of course, Kate. Playing the part of landlady to what seemed like a bunch of teenagers at times was enough to make Polly's cool blonde locks curl at the ends even more than they were prone to do naturally.

'Oh, come on, Kate. Don't you remember what fun Chrissie was at school?' said Jaz, who was looking forward to having someone to swap the latest make-up tips with. Jaz was also eager to update her long curtain of thick black hair inherited from her Indian mother, and Chrissie, a beauty therapist on Virtual Airlines, would be able to fill her in on all the latest looks in New York.

'She'll hog the bathroom and leave her make-up and clothes all over the place,' said Kate grumpily. 'And she'll steal everyone's boyfriend.'
'Polly's the only one among us who's got a boyfriend,' said Laura, looking up from her book on the mating habits of otters. Laura, a TV researcher on a wildlife programme, could always be relied upon to be blunt (rather like her boyish crop). But having never actually met the infamous Chrissie, she had no strong views on her imminent arrival. Instead, she asked, 'Why is she coming to stay, Pol? I thought she was based in New York now.'
'Something to do with a record producer she met on one of her transatlantic flights,' said Polly. 'Apparently he's promised to get her an audition with a new girl band.'
'Oh, for God's sake,' said Kate, who, if the truth be told, was more than a little jealous of Chrissie's thin thighs and exciting life. Her own thighs were not so svelte (thanks to her sweet tooth), while her job as a PA at Crunch Biscuits couldn't be more boring.

Polly, meanwhile, was looking forward to a little distraction (her boyfriend Harry certainly wasn't providing it) and Chrissie was bound to liven things up at 23 Havana Road …

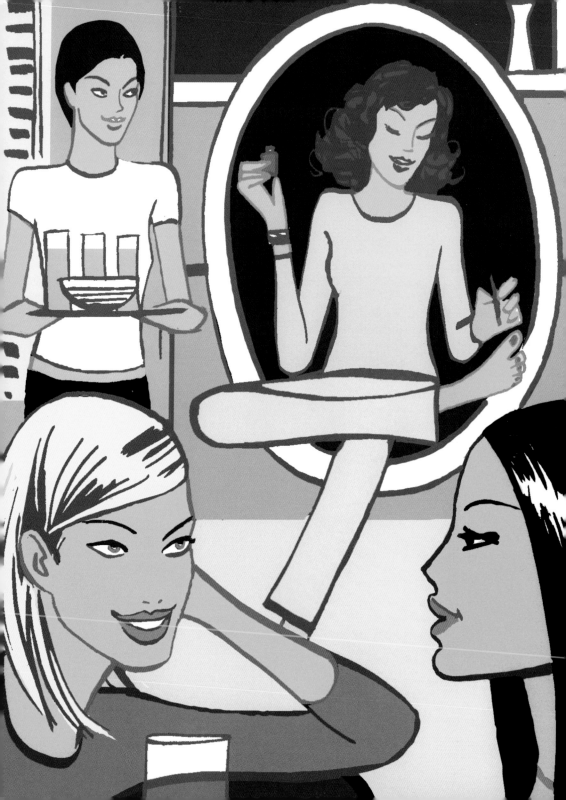

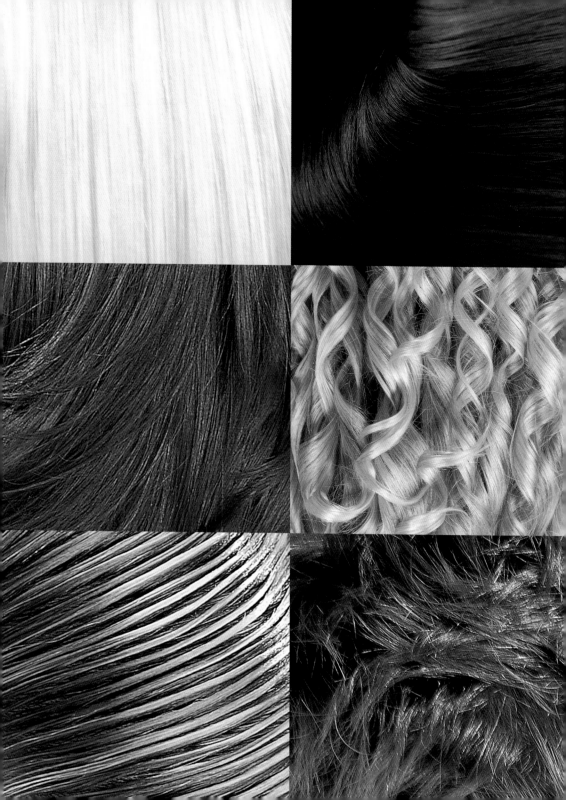

head start

Nothing reflects inner health, vitality and wellbeing quite like a clear complexion, sparkling eyes and – your crowning glory – glossy hair. Beauty comes from within, and if you have an unhealthy diet and lifestyle, your hair – like your skin – will suffer. Tiredness and stress will also wreak havoc on your hair, so modern haircare must be holistic and take into account all aspects of your lifestyle. When you are tense, your scalp tightens and the blood capillaries contract, reducing the quantities of oxygen and nutrients that reach the hair follicles; the production of sweat increases, causing a greasy scalp; and, over prolonged periods of time, stress may even lead to hair loss. A good, relaxing scalp massage can help maintain a healthy head of hair, relieving tension and increasing blood flow, which will, in turn, nourish the root and hair follicle (see page 24 for how to do it).

Clean, shiny hair is a joy to have and head-turning to watch. Yet how often have we been told that our hair is dead, that it is just a build-up of deceased protein cells, strands of keratin which feel no pain when they're cut? This much is true. But hair is also organic in the same way as leather or wood is organic. Just think of how a favourite pair of shoes responds to a good polish, or how a wooden surface shines after a little elbow grease and beeswax. Nourish and condition them and they will shine, 'breathe' and last for years. With the same love and attention, so will your hair. Taking care of your locks is a threefold affair: providing nourishment, treating it with care and using the right products. The simple routines, tips and advice that follow will ensure that you have great salon-style hair every day.

food for thought

The bottom line is that you can't expect to have healthy hair if you eat unhealthily. Whatever products you put onto your tresses, the only real solution is a long-term one that comes from within – a varied diet full of essential vitamins, minerals and other nutrients. Your scalp – where the root and follicle are formed and where 'live' hair grows and develops – forms part of your skin, the largest organ of the body but the last in the queue to receive nourishment from the food we eat (hence the number of skin creams that deliver vitamins and minerals topically). A poor diet means impoverished skin and scalp. If you know your diet is not balanced and you don't want to compromise the health of your hair, then supplement it with a vitamin B complex, antioxidants (including vitamins C, E and beta-carotene), gamma-linolenic acid (GLA), fish oil, linseed oil and the minerals selenium and zinc (see page 26 for more on this). Many chemists sell a good all-round hair and skin supplement.

gently does it

We wouldn't dream of tugging our favourite little black dress on over our head without undoing the zip, or putting our new silk undies in the tumble dryer for 30 minutes on a high heat setting. So why do we think nothing of committing similar crimes to our hair? Imagine your hair to be as precious as a cashmere twinset; treat it accordingly and you will reap the rewards. Brushwork is all-important: poor-quality brushes and combs will scratch the scalp and damage the hair shaft, so don't stint on these (see page 22). Hair is elastic to some extent, but too much pulling will overstretch and ultimately snap it, causing split ends.

no products, no style

Using the right products on your hair could make bad-hair days a thing of the past. The plethora on sale in any chemist, supermarket or salon makes choosing the ones appropriate for your hair type confusing. Slick advertising and packaging makes it even more difficult to get it right. Do you want to go herbal, organic, scientific, fruity or unscented? Will it make your hair bigger, softer, fuller, blonder or seal your split ends? The claims can often be overwhelming – and you just want your hair to look great. The first thing to do is to determine your hair type; once you've got that right, then you can think about the extras. Read on to find out how ...

hair types

Most people tend to wash their hair every day so they probably do not know exactly what hair type they have.

Your hair type is a combination of three factors:

1 The condition of your scalp – is it dry, oily or flaky?

2 The characteristics of your hair – is it fine, frizzy, coarse, curly, wavy, straight or colour-treated?

3 Your environment – do you live in the country or the city? Is your office air-conditioned? Is the climate hot and humid, wet and windy or dry and hot?

normal hair

If your hair is neither prone to oiliness or dryness, you are one of the lucky few to have normal hair. Look after it well with products that keep it clean, conditioned and protected from environmental damage.

combination hair

Five to six hours after washing, hair begins to show signs of oiliness around the root area and yet the ends of the hair remain dry. Oiliness can be caused by overuse of conditioners and styling products, as well as by humidity and pollution.

oily hair

The hair will look oily, dull and 'dirty' along the length of the hair shaft. If you suspect oily hair, make a parting and gently rub your forefinger along your scalp, then rub your thumb and forefinger together. If it feels slippery, you have an oily scalp and overactive sebum glands.

HAIR SNIP

TO CHECK WHICH HAIR TYPE YOU HAVE, WASH YOUR HAIR AS NORMAL AND LET IT DRY NATURALLY. THE NEXT MORNING, BEFORE WASHING YOUR HAIR AGAIN, CHECK FOR SIGNS OF DRYNESS OR OILINESS. YOUR HAIR TYPE WILL CHANGE IF IT CANNOT ADJUST NATURALLY TO CHANGES IN YOUR ENVIRONMENT. IT WILL ALSO PROBABLY CHANGE (BOTH SCALP AND HAIR SHAFT BECOMING DRIER) IF IT IS CHEMICALLY COLOURED OR PERMED.

dry hair

Dry hair will look dull, lifeless and parched; at its worst, it may look fuzzy and straw-like. If you suspect your scalp is dry, look at the white flakes on your shoulders before brushing them away. Small, powdery flakes are often the result of stress, too much alcohol and tiredness. If they are larger, translucent and moist, then it is a case of dandruff, due to overproduction of sebum in the hair follicles, rather than a dry scalp.

hair textures

curly hair

Often the cuticles (the overlapping keratin cells that form hair) do not lie flat on curly hair because of the curved nature of the shaft. This can lead to dull-looking hair and frizz. Overcome this with leave-in conditioners, serums and conditioning sprays.

afro hair

Afro hair is usually dry, brittle and fine. Hydrate the hair with conditioning preparations and massage the scalp gently to promote healthy growth and the production of sebum, the body's natural hair conditioner.

straight hair

The shaft of the hair is straight and, if the hair is in good condition and the cuticles are lying flat (the use of serum can encourage this), straight hair can look super-shiny. In less than ideal conditions, split ends and breakages may be noticeable.

coarse hair

This type of hair can look fuzzy and wiry after shampooing. Use a serum or leave-in conditioner to close and smooth the cuticle and do regular deep-conditioning treatments.

fine hair

Often this type of hair can look lank and lifeless soon after washing. Overconditioning will weigh the hair down, so only use it sparingly. Always use volumizing products especially formulated for fine hair.

chemically treated hair

Although colouring processes are more gentle than ever, some still change the make up of your hair permanently. Give coloured hair extra support by using rehydrating shampoos and conditioners that have been specifically designed for this hair type. Also, check that they contain sunscreen to protect your hair from damage caused by ultraviolet light and keep your colour looking fresh for longer.

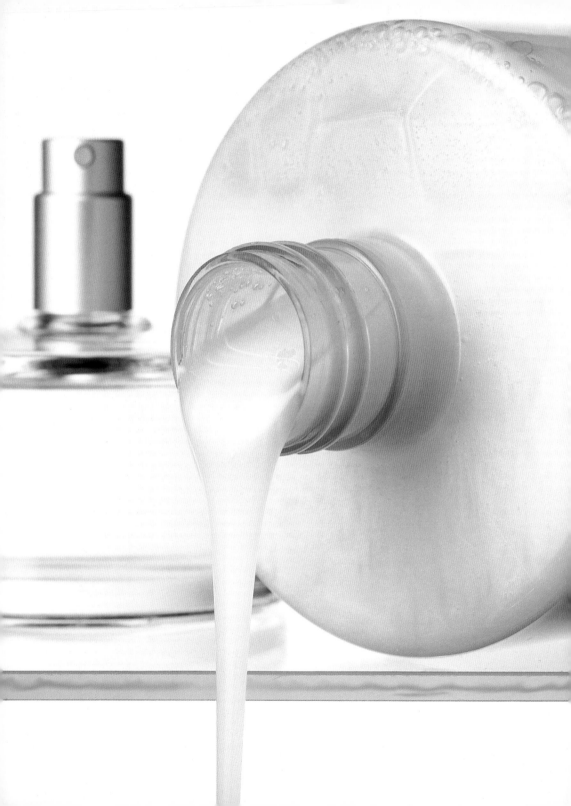

dream routine

Compare your haircare regime to your skincare regime: face – cleanse, tone, moisturize and protect, apply make-up; hair – shampoo, condition and protect, style, finish. A shampoo will gently but effectively cleanse the hair shaft, while a conditioner will moisturize your hair like a good face cream moisturizes your skin. Appropriate styling and finishing products will protect it from heat and oxidation from ultraviolet light and pollution which create dangerous free radicals. There are more benefits to be had by following a four-step haircare regime – shampoo, condition, style, finish – than by relying only on a shampoo.

Few women skip a step in their skincare routine (are there still women who just use soap and water?) because modern products are designed to work together in synergy. The same is true of haircare products. Have you noticed how wonderful your hair looks when you have just been to the hairdressers and had the full treatment of shampoos, conditioners, styling products and finishing spray? Use them all regularly and your hair will become stronger, more flexible and resistant to damage. It's an accumulative effect.

shampoos

Beauty sceptics love to throw scorn on the relative merits of so-called designer shampoos. 'There's no difference between them and washing-up liquid,' is their collective cry. Well, they are wrong. Here's why. There is no denying that a bubble bath might share similar ingredients to a shampoo. But, as with humans whose bodies are made up of 90 per cent water and yet each one is unique, it is the other 10 per cent that makes all the difference. There are many special ingredients added to shampoos that can make hair look and behave as you would like, so experiment to find one that performs best for your hair type. Most modern shampoos are gentle enough to use every day and, in many cases, will actually improve the

condition of hair. It is not necessary to rub your hair like you might your clothes because the surfactant properties of the key ingredients in shampoos allow grime, dust, oil and dirt to lift away from the hair shaft, leaving your hair clean and porous for conditioning.

pH-balanced shampoos

Using a shampoo that is not pH-balanced could damage your hair, so make sure you choose products carefully. Be extremely wary of baby shampoos as some of these are not pH-balanced and are formulated for scalp care rather than for nourishing and cleansing the hair.

dandruff shampoos

Dandruff shampoos have changed dramatically in the past few years. Coal tar, the traditional dandruff cure, has been replaced by new wonder ingredients such as piroctone olamine. The shampoo acts as an exfoliant, as in skincare, to help shed the surplus cells. The best anti-dandruff shampoos include tea tree oil, a natural antiseptic that will not overdry the scalp or damage the hair.

frequently asked questions

Q Is shampooing regularly bad for your hair and will it fade colour?

A No, as long as you use good products that are pH-balanced and contain conditioning agents to seal the cuticle and lock in any colour.

Q Why does my hair feel greasy and my scalp dry after shampooing?

A This comes from not rinsing products away thoroughly. Always rinse the hair until it feels 'squeaky clean' to the touch.

Q Do shampoos, conditioners and styling products cause build-up and if so, what can be done?

A Some products' ingredients can cause a build-up or intolerance. This can be prevented by using a detoxifying shampoo every two weeks, which will also cleanse the hair generally from outside pollution.

the five-step shampoo

1 Thoroughly drench the hair for 30 to 60 seconds before you apply shampoo - you'll need less product and washing will be easier on the hair. Rub a little shampoo between the palms of your hands before smoothing it over the surface of the hair.

2 Gently massage the head, but do not rough up the hair or pull long hair up onto the scalp - it only causes tangles. Long hair will be cleansed as the shampoo washes out with the water.

3 When massaging, use the tips of your fingers, not the palms of your hands. This helps stimulate the scalp and stops you from roughing up the cuticle.

4 Rinse, rinse and rinse again. Poor rinsing results in dull hair and a flaky scalp, caused by dry soap flakes. Finish with an ice-cold rinse. It will close the cuticle and stimulate the scalp, ensuring healthy growth and extra shine.

5 To towel-dry, squeeze and pat the hair dry. Do not rub it too vigorously with the towel as it will rub the hair cuticle up the wrong way.

conditioners

There is much more to conditioners than just their moisturizing ingredients: laws of physics come into play each time you apply one. The positively charged polymers of small and large cationic molecules in the conditioning agents are attracted to and attach themselves to the negatively charged, damaged areas of your hair. In this way, each hair shaft is coated with protective binding and moisturizing ingredients, so conditioners can actually help repair weakened hair. As skincare formulations have become more advanced, so, too, have haircare products, enabling the ingredients to penetrate much deeper into the hair shaft, leaving hair better conditioned and feeling lighter.

hair masks

Deep conditioning treatments and hair masks work on the same principle as everyday conditioners, but because they are left on the hair for longer, they have more time to penetrate the hair shaft. The ingredients are easily absorbed by the hair, so there is no need to leave the treatment on for longer than the recommended time. Use an intensive conditioner or hair mask once a week for super-glossy hair, especially if your tresses are prone to dryness.

leave-in conditioners

These are designed to condition and add shine but do not leave the hair lank which makes them ideal for people with fine, flyaway or difficult-to-manage hair. They are best applied away from the roots.

conditioning tips

Identify your requirements when choosing a conditioner to suit your hair and scalp type, but remember its limitations. No conditioner can replace essential nutrients that are lacking in your diet.

Always read the manufacturer's notes. These provide much more information than ever before, so you shouldn't make the wrong choice.

Once you have applied a hair mask, cover your hair, either with silver foil or clingfilm, both of which lock in the heat and enable the product to penetrate deeper (heat will open the cuticle wider).

Alternatively, drench a towel with hot water and wrap it around your head – you have the bonus of extra heat and the steam will stop the hair drying.

When you rinse off conditioner, finish with a cold blast of water which will close the cuticle, leaving hair glossy and shiny. It will also stimulate blood flow to the scalp, encouraging healthy hair growth.

Key ingredients to look out for in your miracle in a bottle: wheatgerm oil, a natural moisturizer; green tea extract, which helps to retain moisture; and provitamin B5, which enhances gloss.

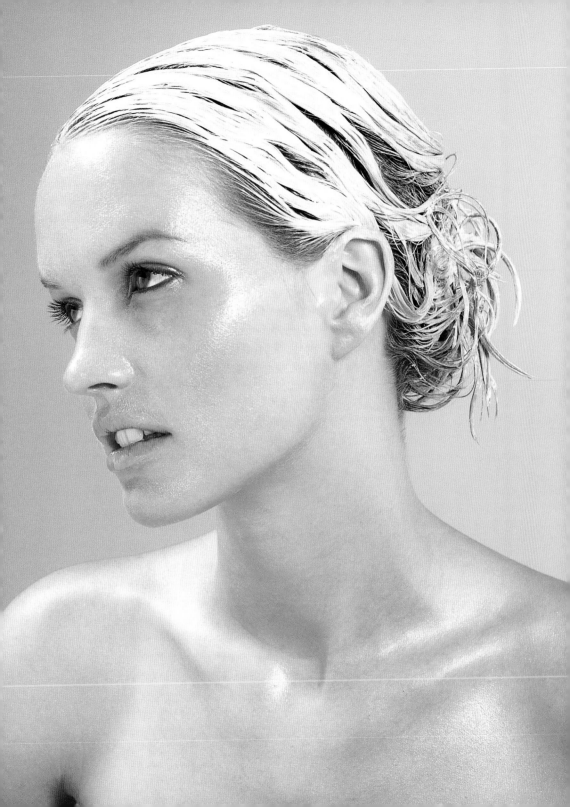

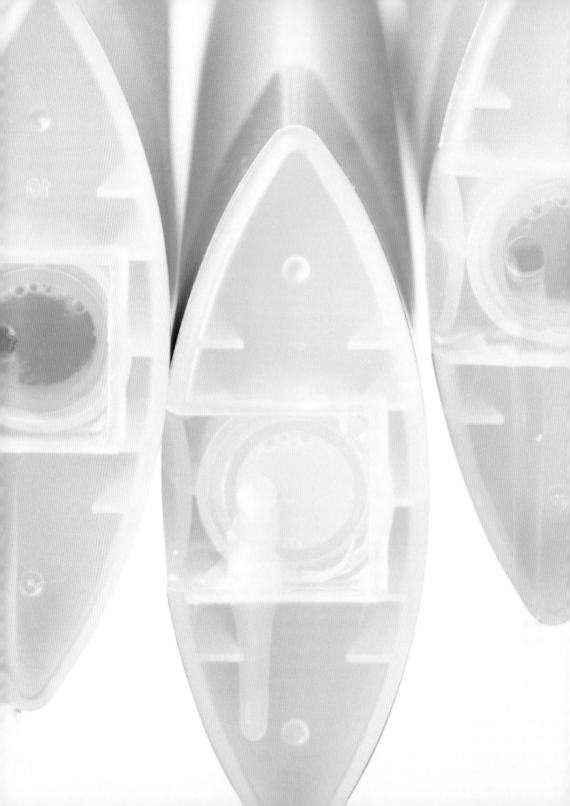

product power

Hair without styling product is like a sandwich without filling; it's the best way to get the most out of your locks. To maintain tip-top condition, use products that are specially formulated for your hair type and that correspond with your shampoo and conditioner. Avoid sticky products, as these tend to create build-up and can ruin the condition and health of your hair. Also, don't overload your hair – it may lose volume and look lank. Forget old myths about styling products; they have improved dramatically in recent years to give added manageability and the control you need to create certain looks. Try out as many products as you can to see which you like, and ask your stylist for advice.

mousse

The light, airy consistency of mousse makes it easy to distribute evenly. The hold factor depends on the resin content – more resins means more lift and hold.

thickening and volumizing sprays

Like mousses, styling sprays use flexible resins to give body and volume. They give an even coverage and tend to be softer and lighter than mousse; the spray application means it can be directed to specific areas, such as a fringe (bangs) or the roots. Both sprays and mousses help combat static. Styling spray is ideal to use on wet hair or as an instant pick-me-up between washes to give great shape and renewed gloss and bounce. It leaves hair looking natural and protects it from heat-styling damage.

gels

These are used to sculpt a style and contain water-soluble resins and silicones that give a firm hold. Depending on the ratio of water to oil in the formula, gels can vary in consistency from ones that set hard after application to those that keep a wet look.

wax

Originally used in Afro haircare, waxes (or pomades) became the hair gels of the 1990s. Used sparingly, waxes (which contain petroleum jelly) give shine and hold down errant strands by virtue of their adhesive consistency.

serum

The latest hair styling innovation is a volatile silicone which imparts brilliant shine to hair with none of the heaviness of wax. It must be used very sparingly, otherwise hair looks oily. The spray versions tend to be heavier and can't be controlled as well as pump-action serums.

straighteners

These temporarily close down the cuticle to achieve a smooth, sleek finish. Use one in conjunction with a straightening blow-dry (see page 61) and Jennifer Aniston's look could be yours.

always read the label

There are key ingredients to look out for when choosing the right products for your hair type. There is no need to be blinded by science for a moment longer – all will be revealed:

Amino acids act as humectants, drawing moisture into the hair.

Cationic ingredients are positively charged molecules (usually polymers) that are attracted to damaged areas of the hair shaft and lock on to smooth and repair.

Green tea extract is an antioxidant that combats free radical damage and improves hair health.

Panthenol or Provitamin B5 penetrates the hair shaft to improve strength, moisture and shine.

Polymers give bounce and manageability. Water-soluble silicones and dimethicones coat the hair to smooth the cuticle and add shine.

Vitamin E, or tocopherol, is a protective antioxidant that slows down oxidation caused by pollution, smoking, chlorine and UV exposure.

Wheatgerm oil moisturizes the hair and also decreases static.

brushwork

It seems such a simple and obvious thing – using the right tool for the job – and yet few do it. The choice of brush can affect how fast your hair dries, how smooth it is and how much volume you can create. Good-quality bristles protect hair from splitting and stretching, making styling and combing easier and painless, while poor-quality brushes and combs will scratch the scalp and damage the hair shaft. When choosing a brush, always check that the teeth and bristles are smooth.

paddle brush
Broad and rectangular, it smooths hair and works best on long, straight styles. The rubber cushioning on the paddle ensures extra-smooth, static-free hair.

roller and curling brushes
Used with a hairdryer, roller and curling brushes become mobile curlers and achieve volume. Some have a metal barrel that conducts heat from the dryer to reduce drying times. These can be detached from the handle to form a roller, which is ideal for creating long-lasting volume. If your hair has a tendency to be static, then lightly spray the metal barrel with hairspray.

volumizing brushes
These are the ones with an 'open' head and fewer bristles or teeth than most other brushes. The holes work like air vents to circulate warm air from a hairdryer and increase volume and bounce.

smoothing brushes
An essential day-to-day brush that often has a rubber cushion holding the bristles, helping to counter static electricity. It is good to have a mix of natural and nylon bristles – nylon will grip, while natural will smooth.

tail combs
Used for sectioning hair when blow-drying or setting, they are the only way to create a perfect parting.

fork combs
These 'open' up curls and separate kinky, wavy hair.

fine and medium combs
Both of these are used for backcombing and delicate detangling, but are best used by a hairdresser.

wide-tooth combs
Use these to comb conditioner through wet hair.

brushstrokes
Hair is elastic to some extent, but harsh brushing will overstretch and ultimately break the hair.

1 Always brush your hair before shampooing to massage the scalp, help loosen dead skin cells and detangle any knots (the hair becomes more fragile and thus more difficult to detangle when wet).

2 Always brush from the tips up, not from the roots down. This is the best way to detangle hair.

3 To remove a tangle, comb from the base of the tangle to hair tips, working upwards slowly.

4 Once hair is tangle-free, brush from the roots to the tips to distribute sebum along the hair shaft and increase its natural shine.

5 Ignore the '100 brushstrokes a day' maxim. Too much brushing will overstimulate sebum production and increase the chances of oily hair, breakages and split ends. In the Victorian times when this old-wives' tale was coined, 100 strokes a day was a good way of preventing hair lice from multiplying because it destroyed the eggs and damaged the insects. Yuck!! Times have changed and so should our grooming habits. Rapunzel had more time on her hands than you.

6 Keep brushes and combs clean and free from stray hairs and product build-up. Add a little shampoo to lukewarm water and soak them for about five minutes, then leave to dry naturally.

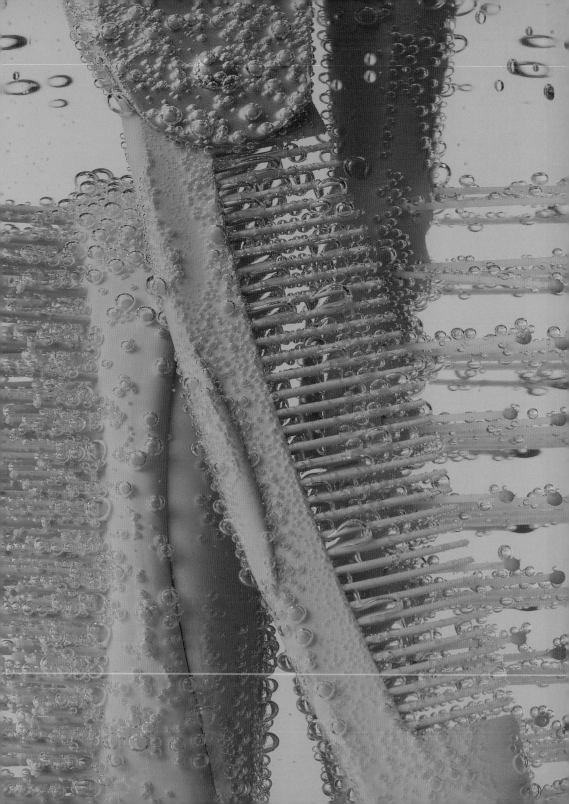

inside, outside

In a perfect world we would all be calm, collected and look the picture of health. Unfortunately, though, all too often we are subject to stress, but how we deal with it determines how well we cope and, ultimately, how good we look. Taking supplements, exercising and allowing time to eat well, sleep well and relax will not make your life go more smoothly, but it will give your inner resources an extra boost that will help you manage stress and still have enough energy left to keep your inner light shining brightly.

expect the unexpected

From relatively minor disruptions like the washing machine flooding to more serious problems of health and demands from your work and family, life is full of situations beyond our control. Inevitably, this means we often have to change the best-laid plans at the last moment and adapt accordingly. When we are fit and healthy we are more able to deal with problems and to respond more effectively to them.

don't be too harsh on yourself

Good habits are easy to break and no one is immune to temptation. If your willpower isn't as strong as you'd like, maybe you are expecting too much of yourself. Reconsider your goals. Few people manage to eat a perfectly balanced diet or keep up an exercise routine all of the time.

learn to compromise

We all lead busy, busy lives and free time has become a luxury. If a few microwave meals are a way of spending precious time with your family, then so be it. But you don't have time to relax? You don't have to be in a yoga class to practise slow, deep breathing – do it while driving home in your car or while sitting on the bus.

get as much help as you can

Develop a support system of your favourite products, dietary supplements and pampering treats that you can use to nurture your sense of wellbeing. Keep to hand a list of the numbers of good health, beauty and alternative therapists so that booking a reflexology appointment becomes as easy as dialling out for a takeaway.

stressed hair

When you are worried and stressed, the first part of the body to become tense is the shoulders. When the neck and shoulders are constricted, the supply of oxygen and blood to the scalp is inhibited. Inevitably, your hair becomes stressed, too, and the signs are a flaky scalp, dull hair and, eventually, hair loss. When you are stressed, your nails and hair are the first to be ignored by your body's natural vitamin distribution process – and this is also true for pregnant women. It is absolutely essential to replace lost minerals and vitamins, both internally and externally.

1 Massage the scalp and learn to relax. It relieves tension and increases blood flow which nourishes the root and hair follicle. Gently work your fingers around your head, massaging all the time. Start at the perimeter of the head and work inwards, making sure your fingers never leave the scalp.

2 A flaky scalp can be due to dehydration – especially after too much alcohol – so take a bath to unwind, rather than reaching for the wine bottle, and always drink at least eight large glasses of water every day.

3 Consider supplementing your diet with vitamins and minerals.

4 Eat your greens. Green vegetables have a high iron content that will encourage the growth of healthy hair.

5 Eat oily fish. The oils encourage the flow of sebum, thus giving flexibility to the hair.

6 Essential oils are good for wellbeing and can also benefit the scalp and hair when a few drops are diluted in vegetable oil or warm water. Rose absolut is moisturizing; tea tree and eucalyptus have antiseptic properties which are soothing for a dry, tight scalp; and lavender is supremely relaxing.

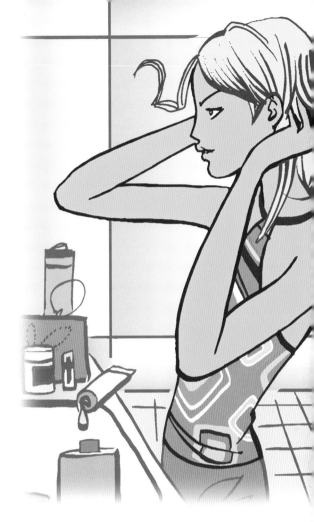

Having spent the night on a mattress on Polly's floor, Chrissie feels underwhelmed, jet-lagged and out of sorts. She didn't get the red-carpet treatment she'd been expecting – her sleeping arrangements left a lot to be desired and where was she meant to be hanging up her (extensive) wardrobe? Standing in the bathroom under the glare of a very unflattering light, she realizes that she is experiencing the mother of all bad-hair days. Chrissie's fine flyaway locks are looking fluffy, fuzzy and lank. Her job as beauty therapist on Virtual

... chrissie's frazzled-hair crisis

Airlines has caused big problems on the static front. All those long, carpeted corridors at Heathrow, the nylon upholstery and the fetching beret she's forced to wear ensure that sparks fly every time she brushes her hair. It's no wonder she's failed to pull the handsome dot.com entrepreneur who commutes to New York every week; each time she gives him

a back massage he complains of static shocks. And now this. She looks like a cross between an ageing rock star and Dougal from *The Magic Roundabout*. Working frantically through the contents of the bathroom cabinet, she experiments with every hair product she can lay her hands on in an attempt to groom her sorry, straggling

strands – but to no avail. It finally dawns on Chrissie that no amount of serum is going to solve her hair crisis. What her stressed-out mane really needs is some back-to-basic haircare – the magic H_2O (at least 1 litre a day) and some dietary supplements like vitamin B and C (a balanced diet is not one of Chrissie's strong points).

fringe benefits

The debate about whether or not to take supplements is on-going. Many doctors and dieticians believe that a balanced diet, containing plenty of fresh fruit and vegetables, should provide all the nutrients the body needs to function efficiently and at its optimum. However, the lifestyle that many of us lead means that we are frequently under stress and exposed to toxins – both from an intake of caffeine, nicotine, alcohol and overprocessed food, and also from ultraviolet rays, pollution and radiation from office equipment – which can deplete our bodies' stores of essential nutrients.

supplements for hair, skin and nails

Beta-carotene is an antioxidant that is converted in the body to form vitamin A.

Omega-3 provides essential fatty acids.

Starflower oil is a rich source of an essential fatty acid, gamma linolenic acid (GLA), which acts as a building block for healthy skin and hormone balance.

Selenium is a mineral needed for the action of many antioxidant enzymes.

Vitamin B complex promotes healthy hair and skin and supports the central nervous system.

Vitamin C is an antioxidant that destroys harmful free radicals caused by pollution.

Zinc is a mineral that is essential for the proper functioning of over 100 enzymes.

warning

Supplements are virtually non-toxic, so there is no real safety issue. A good multivitamin, multimineral and an antioxidant formula is ideal, but if in doubt, ask a doctor, dietician or pharmacist for advice and always follow the manufacturer's dosage instructions. If you are experiencing any serious problems with your hair, consult a doctor for advice.

supplements for stress

Beta-carotene, selenium and vitamins C and E with zinc work together as antioxidants to disarm damaging free radicals caused by stress.

Bilberry helps prevent the premature death of body cells.

Calcium and magnesium deficiencies are common in highly stressed individuals and can result in anxiety, fear and even hallucinations.

Dong quai supports the kidneys, central nervous system and the adrenal glands, which are among the most susceptible organs to stress.

Gamma-aminobutric acid (GABA) acts as a tranquillizer and is important for proper brain function.

Gingko biloba aids brain function and circulation.

Hops help to ease nervousness, restlessness and stress, and also decrease the desire for alcohol.

Kava kava relaxes the mind as well as the body.

L-Tyrosine is an effective sleeping aid, which is also good for depression.

Valerian is another powerful sleeping aid when taken at bedtime and it also helps ease stress-related headaches.

Vitamin B complex, plus extra vitamin B6 (pyridoxine), B12 and B5 (panothenic acid) are necessary for health and the proper functioning of the nervous system; B5, in particular, is an anti-stress vitamin needed by the thymus gland.

Vitamin C with bioflavonoids is essential for the functioning of the adrenal gland, which produces anti-stress hormones.

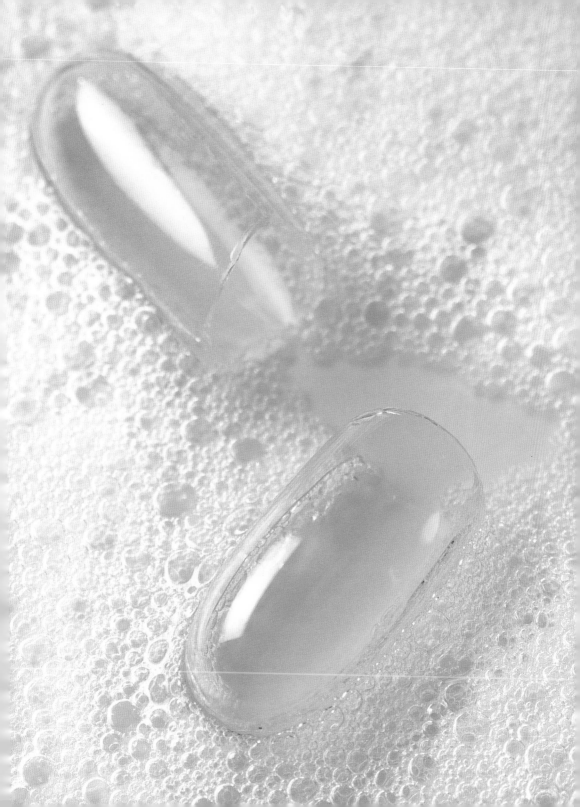

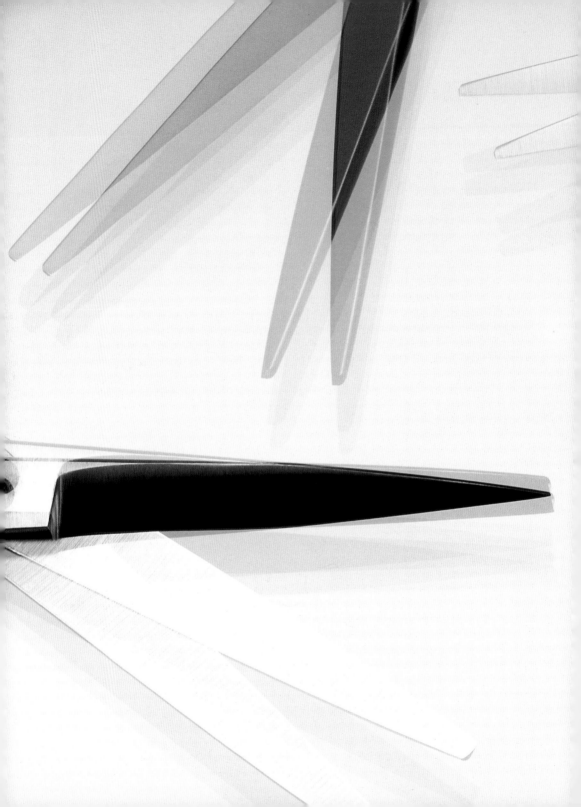

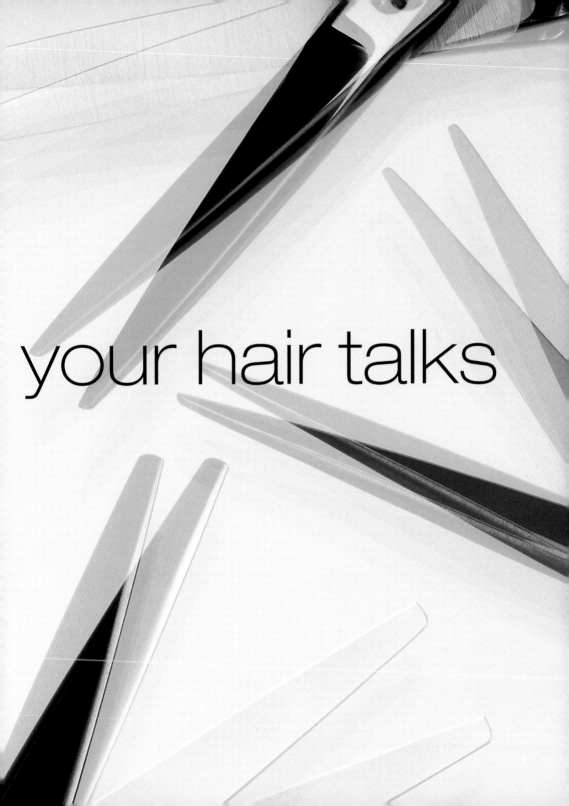

your hair talks

chrissie comes to town

'I can't tell you how thrilled I am to be here,' said Chrissie, gliding elegantly into the sitting room, bare-footed and bare-legged, save for a silver chain around her ankle that jangled as she moved. The girls were lined up on the (once) cream-coloured sofa, marvelling at how glamorous their new house guest looked. Despite the fact that it was Sunday morning, Chrissie was wearing full make-up, artfully contrived to look as if she was wearing none at all.

'So I've brought each of you a little present from the Big Apple,' she was saying, dipping into a big honey-coloured leather bag that Jaz instantly recognized as a designer label that you had to join a 12-month waiting-list to own. 'For Polly, my gracious hostess … something sexy to go under all those deathly boring navy-blue suits that you have to wear to work.' Chrissie handed over a little parcel of shell-pink tissue paper containing a scarlet silk camisole with black lace trim. 'I thought it might spice things up a little with Harry,' she added. Polly blushed the same colour as the camisole. It would take more than this to spice things up with Harry, her boyfriend since college. He was a nice enough bloke, but these days he seemed to get more turned on by share prices than by Polly's choice of lingerie. Their relationship had gone a little flat, to say the least. It was a good job that she had flirtatious e-mails from her colleague in New York to look forward to. At least 'cyber-Simon', as she called him, was adding a little fizz to her life. 'And for you, Kate … a new cellulite cream,' Chrissie was saying. 'I've heard

from girlfriends who have cellulite that it really works.' Kate glowered as Chrissie handed over the tube of Fat-busting Miracle Lotion. Jaz, meanwhile, was thrilled with her set of brain-boosting nail polishes containing ginkgo biloba – 'absorbed through the nail bed to improve brain function' – and oblivious to the implied insult. 'And Laura, I think this scent is just the ticket for you. It smells … well, very feminine,' said Chrissie, in what was clearly a dig at Laura's tomboy style. Laura, who never wore perfume, stifled the urge to laugh as she eyed the blurb on the label: 'Fatal: The scent that spells instant attraction'. Love her or loathe her – and Laura hadn't made her mind up yet – there was no denying that Chrissie was a blast.

'Now girls, the good news is that Steve, the record producer I told you about, has invited me to the opening of Shaft, a new bar in Soho, on Saturday night,' Chrissie continued, 'and I've managed to get you all on the guest list.'
'Thanks, but no thanks. I've already got plans,' lied Kate, who would rather boil in oil than spend an evening with Chrissie.
'Count me in,' declared Jaz enthusiastically (she was already painting her toenails orange).
'I'm game,' said Laura. 'What about you, Pol?'
'I'd love to, but I'm flying to New York on Saturday afternoon for business and I'll be away for the rest of the week,' replied Polly, who could hardly contain her excitement at the prospect of finally meeting Simon, her sexy (she hoped) cyber-suitor.

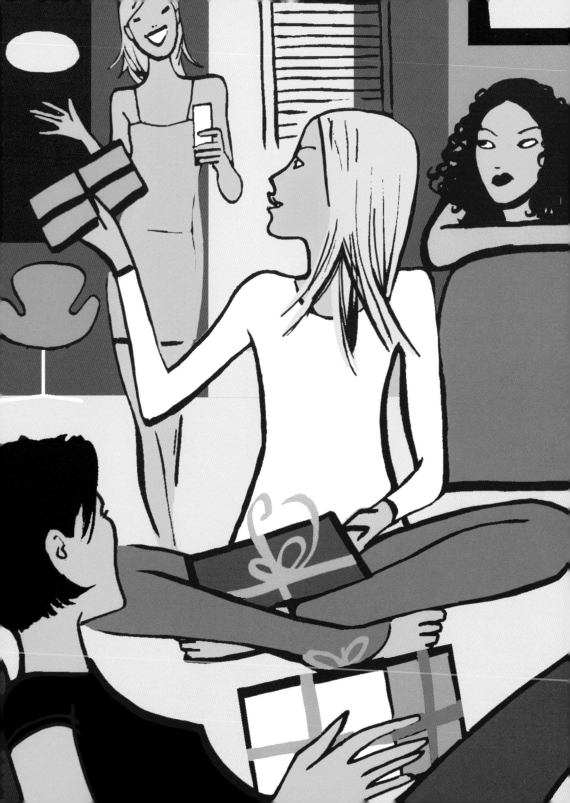

cut it

There are no limitations to your choice of style or cut. Modern fashion and beauty tells us that anything goes: all that matters is that you feel happy and confident with your look. If you have a long, sloping jaw, traditional thinking would tell you to avoid a short gamine cut, but if you like it and have the confidence to wear it, the chances are you will pull it off beautifully. Just look at all those quirky models who don't fit the perfectly proportioned, blonde-haired, blue-eyed aesthetic. But if you don't feel brave enough to throw caution to the wind, here are few guidelines that will guarantee that a cut suits your face and flatters your features in a more classical manner.

face shape

The best way to determine your face shape is by doing the mirror trick (see page 34). Alternatively, get a photo taken or rely on your hairdresser to define your profile. Certain features can be minimized or emphasized by a hairstyle. A prominent nose or chin can be countered by a fringe (bangs). An angular jawbone means you can wear gamine Audrey Hepburn cuts and crops, while a long, sloping jawbone doesn't always work with short hair.

Remember that your face shape changes with age. Your jaw will inevitably grow less defined and your complexion less radiant and smooth as you grow older. The good news is that a clever cut and colour can make you look younger and feel better. Don't get stuck in a rut, repeating the same hairstyle time and time again; keep moving with the times. After all, what suits you at 18 is unlikely to look good when you are 30. Nothing will date you faster than make-up and a haircut, and yet nothing is quite so simple to change.

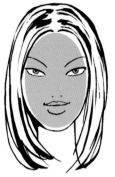

oval face

This classic shape can take any look. With this in mind, use your hairstyle to create an illusion of the perfect oval by balancing out the proportions.

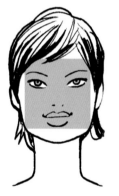

heart-shaped

The narrowing of the face can be countered with the extra volume of a layered bob, which flicks outwards at chin level.

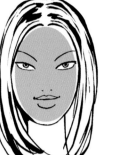

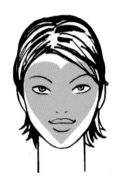

square face

Soften up the edges with a style that breaks up the symmetry. Play with off-centre partings, graduated layers and soft curls.

round face

Soft, feathery cuts with layers coming forward onto the face look stylish and sophisticated and also slim down a fuller face.

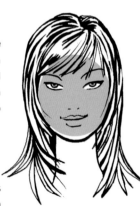

long face

A fringe (bangs) disguises a long forehead, while a chin- or shoulder- length style adds volume and broadens the face.

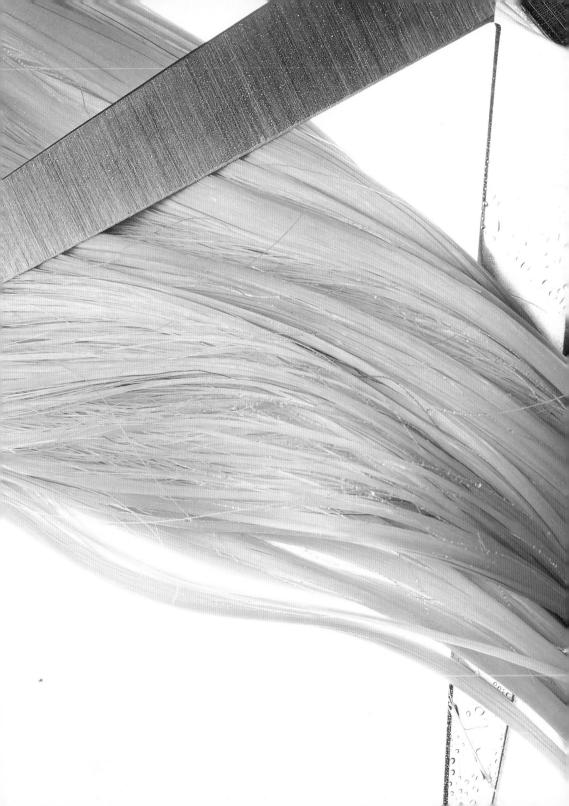

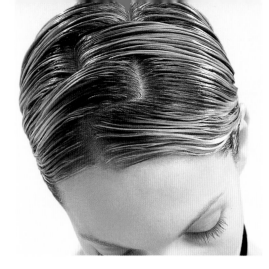

parting company

Creating a new parting is the quickest and cheapest way to update a style and change your look and face shape. Each season, one type of parting dominates the fashion shows – from the zigzag to the deep, side parting just above the ear. For a long time only centre partings would do. Use a tail comb to experiment. Hold it by the teeth at a low angle and use the handle to part the hair. Keep the tip in contact with the scalp to get the most control.

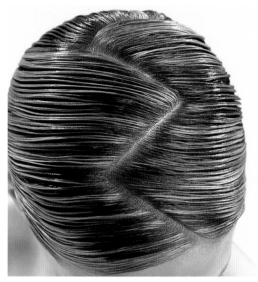

body proportion

As well as considering your hair type and face shape, a good hairdresser will also take into account your body shape, proportions and size when consulting you about a restyle. This is why it is important that he or she sees you to discuss your ideas before you are sitting in a chair, shrouded in a gown and with your hair wrapped up in a towel on top of your head.

Very long, flowing hair on a short body frame will foreshorten the body even more; conversely, a short, gamine crop will not work well on a body that is broad-framed and tall. Big-volume curly shoulder-length hair on a short, plump torso will just accentuate width; while a short, spiky cut on a tall person can be intimidating.

how to determine face shape

1 Stand in front of your mirror, face on.

2 Using your hands, pull all your hair right away from your face.

3 Take a lipstick (not your favourite) and, at arm's length, draw around the outline of your face on the mirror.

4 Like it or not, what you are left with is your face shape.

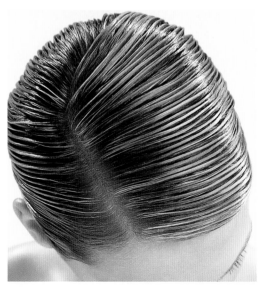

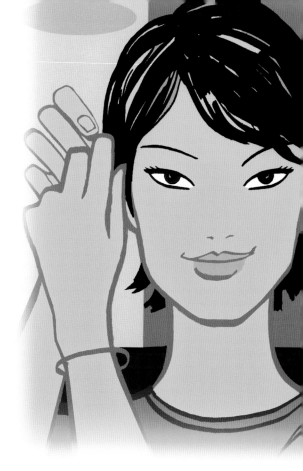

Laura is quite the antithesis of Jaz. That's not to say she doesn't care about her image – she always manages to look effortlessly cool – she just can't be doing with Jaz's overwhelming 'girliness'. Listening to her and Chrissie prattle on last night

… laura's restyle

about the best pink nail polish and where to buy the prettiest handkerchief tops had almost driven her to commit a violent act. Laura has a much more pragmatic approach to beauty. She loves to work out and has had the same boyish crop – quick to wash and dry after her gym sessions – since she started at university in Manchester, which is well over five years ago now. She knows that it's definitely time

for a restyle (her mind was well and truly made up when she heard someone refer to her as 'him' – she did have her back turned, but nevertheless it was not a moment she wants to revisit). Laura books an appointment with her hairstylist who, after a lengthy discussion – after all, this is not a decision to be taken lightly – enthusiastically cuts and restyles her hair. The end result gives her more height on the crown, a soft, wispy

fringe (bangs) on her forehead and light flick-outs on the nape of her neck. The crowning glory, however, is that this new style disguises her large forehead and shortens her long face (not that she would ever admit to minding about these features) – amazing how a cut can change the shape of your face. Laura strides out of the salon with a spring in her step, secretly hoping that the assistant producer in Current Affairs will sit up and take notice.

the cutting edge

A good haircut should make you feel fantastic. It should increase your confidence, make you feel sexy, taller, slimmer, more powerful, and, most importantly, it should reflect your personality. Styled in the right way, a haircut can even act as an instant 'facelift', helping to detract attention from areas of the face that show signs of ageing and, instead, highlight your most flattering features, perhaps great bone structure or beautiful eyes. A good cut will give your entire look a new lease of life – while a little colour on your tresses will make it look thicker and glossier, too (see page 42). Hair is usually the first thing to be altered when a woman is making a major life change – perhaps a new career direction or at the beginning (or end) of a relationship. A visit to the hairdresser's for a spot of pampering or reinvention is also a sure-fire way to lift a bad mood. Once you've found the right hairstyle, everything else falls into place. Whatever the reason and whatever the style, always have a trim every six weeks to avoid split ends and help maintain condition and manageability.

cutting considerations

There are three essential points to consider before embarking on any change of image:

1 Be realistic. How much time do you really want to spend on your hair every day? Also, how much time have you realistically got? If you choose a style that requires time you are not happy to put in, you will never get the look you want.

2 Straight, curly, dark or blonde, wavy or wispy, make the most of what you've got. Hair always looks its best when it is in fabulous condition and has a fantastic cut.

3 Use your ammunition! Products are essential daily tools for achieving gloss, body and manageability on all hair types. Experiment a little and learn which products suit your hair best and how to use them.

the long and the short of it

Long, romantic, tumbling tresses remain a classic look and a favourite with the opposite sex. To counter the hippie 'curtain' effect and make your hair seem less heavy, as well as keep locks in excellent condition, go for a layered cut. This will add shape around your face to give a defined and confident style. With well-shaped layers, hair will not fall too heavily across the face. But be warned: there's nothing worse than straggly, uncared-for, 'rat tail' hair snaking down your back, so don't bother growing it if you don't want to spend time brushing, washing, drying and styling it.

With its mix of modernity and femininity, short hair can be extremely sexy. It is a great option for women who want a strong, feminine image, a personal signature, yet a low-maintenance style. Short, sassy, sexy styles are on the increase – think Meg Ryan, Gwyneth Paltrow and Cameron Diaz. Casual or glamorous, layers help to define texture and volume, giving the hair greater depth and making styling simple.

going for the chop

Ultimately, whether you opt for a long or short style, determining your face shape, hair type and texture will help you to find the most flattering cut for you. Once you have this basic information to work with, you can then adapt catwalk styles or ideas from the pages of beauty magazines to create an individual look. The key thing to remember is that the face shape should trigger off the hairstyle. In the same way as a beautiful frame enhances a picture, if you've got the right hairstyle for your face shape, then your whole face will look prettier and fresher, your eyes will stand out and your good features will be emphasized. Enjoy your hair's own unique style and, with the advice of your hairdresser, select a style to enhance what you've already got. If you try to alter your natural hair too much, you may end up compromising on the condition of your hair and become a slave to a high-maintenance look in the process.

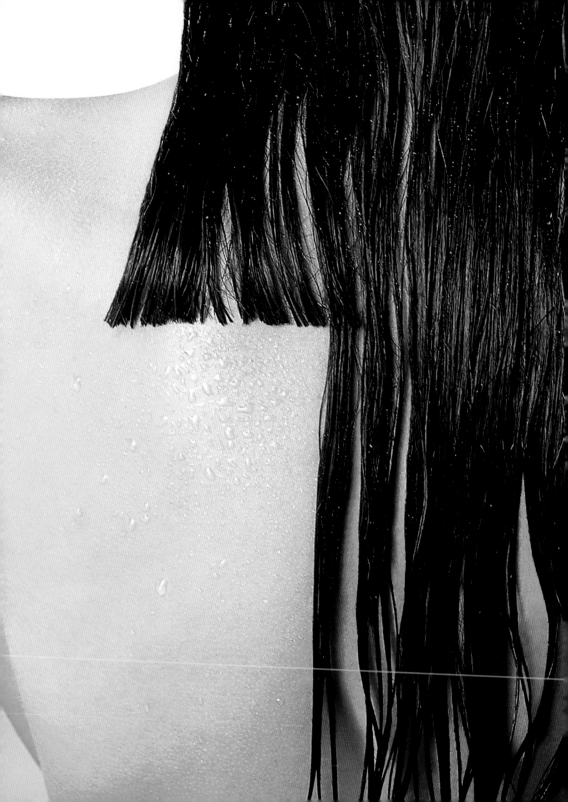

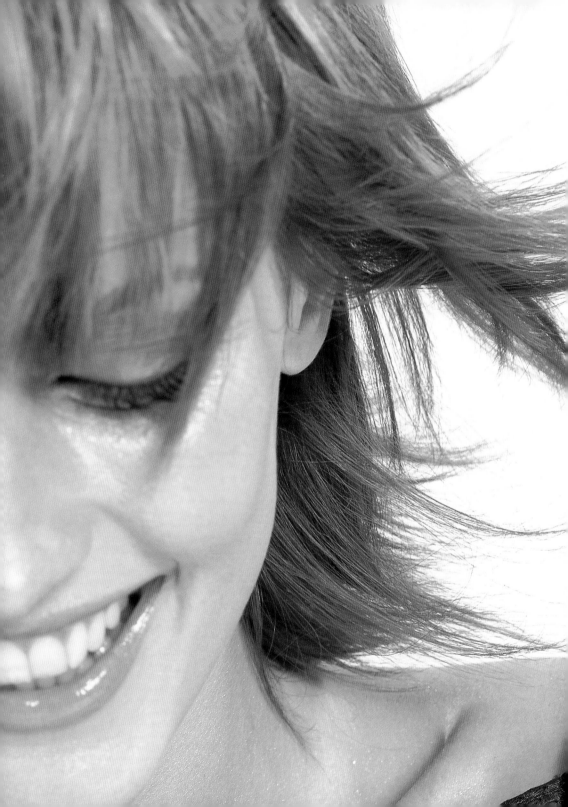

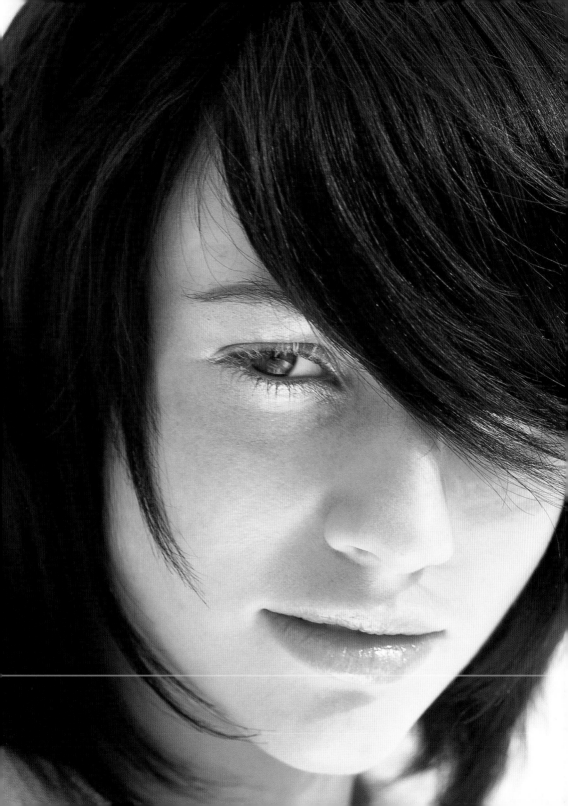

your hairdresser

Finding a hairstylist with whom you 'click' is like any other relationship – although it's unlikely you'd ask a friend to make you look and feel like a groovier version of your favourite actress. You need chemistry, you need trust and you need to be able to convey your ideas in such a way that they can be easily interpreted. If you are considering a radical cut but don't have a hairdresser you trust, book in a few blow-drys at different salons. Mention your ideas to the stylist looking after you and decide with whom you feel most at ease. All good salons offer a free consultation, but having a blow-dry will allow you to experience how a stylist works, rather than just listen to their suggestions. Apart from anything else, visiting a salon should be a pleasurable experience. You want to feel pampered and relaxed, confident in the knowledge that when you walk out you are going to look and feel like a million dollars, not nervous and edgy, wishing you'd brought a paper bag with you.

Recommendations from friends are a good way of finding a reputable stylist, but we are all subjective in our choices, and one person's dream stylist could be another's idea of hell. If you see someone with a haircut you like, ask them who did it. After all, you wouldn't hesitate to question where someone got their stunning kitten heels that you liked the look of, now would you?

the consultation

Taking along a picture of a cut or colour you like is a good starting point and avoids confusion. Compile a 'look book' – a scrapbook or folder where you keep tear sheets from magazines of styles you like, as well as photographs of yourself when you had a particularly good cut or colour. It's also useful to show your stylist pictures of looks that you really dislike. A picture is a good way of understanding one another's vocabulary – for you, titian may mean coppery golden tints; for your stylist it may mean gingery red tones. However, do not expect to look like the person in the picture – sadly for us, there is only one Rachel, one Meg and one Gwyneth.

reworkings and rewards

If you don't like a cut or style, be honest and tell your stylist. They would much prefer to rework it and sort it out for you, rather than have you leave disappointed. Conversely, if you really like a cut or receive a lot of compliments on a style, give the stylist that feedback. Everyone responds to praise and likes to know when a cut or style performs well.

If you are happy with the stylist's work, then tip, but don't feel uneasy if you can't afford to tip heftily. Ask any hairdresser and they are thrilled if they receive a thank-you card or see a customer leave the salon looking genuinely happy. Equally, if you buy a bottle of the shampoo, conditioner or styling product that your stylist has used, this indicates that you want to re-create the look again at home.

hairdressers' translation service

Choppy This is the result when hair has been cut using a texturizing method – for example, razor-cutting to give a 'choppy finish'.

Feathery Using a razor to cut hair instead of scissors. This creates a much more random finish, leaving the hair more dishevelled and giving that lived-in look.

Flick-outs This involves blow-drying the hair so that it flicks outwards at the ends to create volume and width, instead of blow-drying the hair under, which is a more traditional look.

Texturizing A method of cutting using tools such as a razor, clippers or texturizing scissors. These are like ordinary cutting scissors, but one blade is serrated, enabling the stylist to reduce weight evenly throughout the cut.

Volume To build hair and add life, volume can be temporary or permanent.

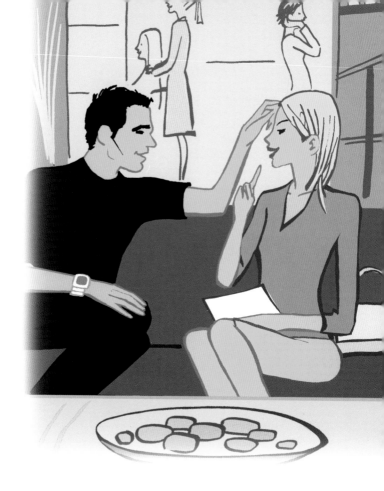

... polly's hair therapy

Chrissie's arrival has precipitated a bit of a *crise* in Polly's life. She takes one look at Chrissie's tardis-like suitcase – the copious contents of which are now strewn across her bedroom floor – and compares her stiff power suits and boring basics with Chrissie's endless supply of skimpy T's in every shade of pink and purple, bead-fringed capri pants and flirty, diaphanous skirts. And was that a diamanté, heart-shaped body jewel stuck to her sensible beige carpet? Polly decides there is nothing else for it but to book a day at her favourite hair and beauty spa for a bit of top-to-toe pampering. She's been 'seeing' Charles for years – he always has a knack of understanding exactly what she wants, and has a chair-side manner to die for – not to mention the great haircuts. After lots of hair chat (so much better than therapy), Polly decides to have her shoulder-length blonde hair lightly layered, which will soften her face and groove up her look. Best of all, it can be zooped up with products for that hip rock-chick look – although the latter probably won't go down too well with the suits on the top floor! Polly feels fantastic. Harry won't recognize her – on second thoughts, he probably won't even notice.

colour coding

Colour adds sheen, gloss, texture, thickness, depth and life to your hair and can be used either to enhance your natural hair colour or to explore a different side of your personality and change your image. Never be afraid to experiment, especially when you have a trusted stylist with whom you feel safe enough to be a little more daring. A good colourist will work with your skin tone and personality to create an effect that suits your style and boosts your confidence.

hue are you?

An experienced colourist is able to determine quickly whether you are a 'whisper', 'talk' or 'scream' type of customer – in other words, whether you would be more comfortable with a few lowlights in your mousey brown hair or whether you are an extrovert who will feel perfectly at ease with a white-blonde crop. Often a customer profile questionnaire is used as part of a two-way discussion between stylist and customer to establish which colours will go best with your personality, as well as which will suit your complexion.

the home colour zone

Use the colour chart on pages 46–7 to work out whether you are a 'warm' or 'cool' customer. This will help you determine which hair colours will best enhance your skin tone (see right).

1 Stand in front of a mirror in good (preferably natural) light, holding the colour chart just underneath your chin.

2 Slowly move it from left to right and back again and observe which colour tones are the most flattering to your complexion.

3 Repeat the process a few times and ask the opinion of a friend.

natural mixes

The colour of your hair should be from the same family (warm or cool) as your skin tone. If you have very pale skin, any colour will look good; if you have pink skin, avoid reds and warm golds; if your skin has yellow tones, favour deep reds and avoid golds; those with black or olive skin should stay dark, adding richness and depth with lowlights. Use the following guide to help determine what hair colour will best suit your complexion and colouring, or try on wigs or hairpieces.

warm

Eyes: brown, hazel, green or dark brown.

Skin: freckles, golden beige, bronze or golden brown.

Hair: golden or strawberry blonde, golden brown or auburn, chestnut or dark brown.

cool

Eyes: grey-blue, grey-brown or rose-brown.

Skin: beige, rose-brown or cocoa.

Hair: ash blonde, ash brown, beige blonde, black, burgundy or plum.

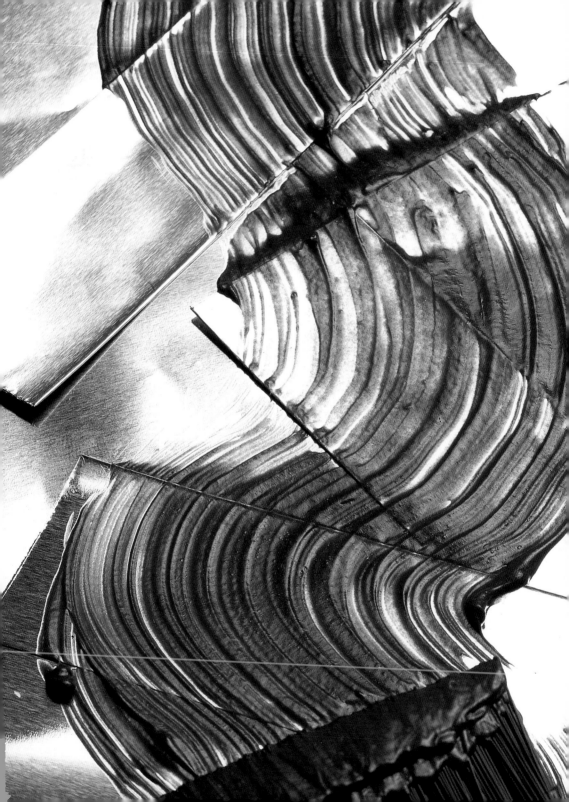

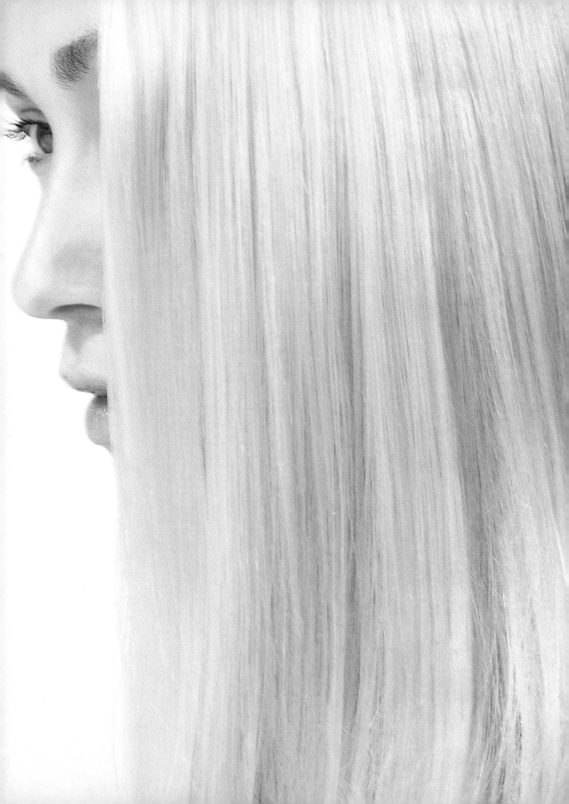

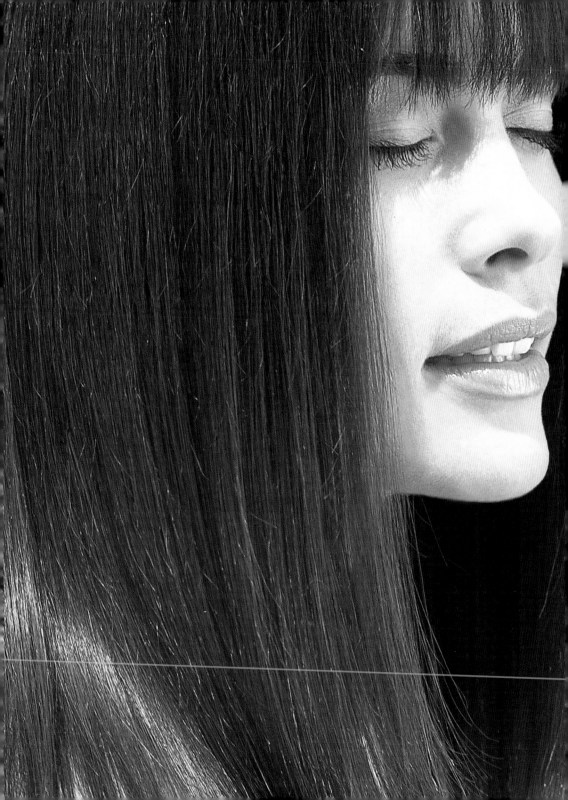

colour glossary

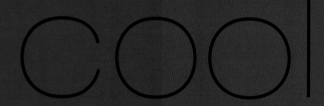

semi-permanent colour

These are vegetable-based dyes that penetrate slightly into the hair, then simply wash away. They last for about 12 washes. You can go only darker or warmer than your natural colour.

highlights

With highlighting, strands of hair are placed in foils and dyed a lighter shade than your natural colour. Bold strands create a strong effect, while fine pieces give a more natural look. As the dye is permanent, the roots will need retouching when the highlights grow out.

permanent colour

These dyes can improve the condition of the hair while adding colour. You can go lighter, darker or change the tone completely. The colour does not appear artificial, no matter how vivid the tone. This process can be carried out as a full head or as pieces of colour.

lowlights

With lowlights, strands of hair are placed in foils and dyed a darker shade than your natural hair colour. The dye is permanent. This is a very good method of adding depth and tone to dull hair – you can be as subtle or as bright as you want.

colour wash

Change your look for the weekend with a colour wash. This temporary colour is available as a coloured mousse or setting lotion and will last for just one wash. Also known as vegetable colours, these are excellent for refreshing faded colour and can be used as a conditioning treatment.

tone on tone

This technique blends white hair and adds tone and shine. It will not lighten hair, but gives it sheen and life. Tone-on-tone lasts between four and six weeks. This can also be used within creative-colour techniques to give subtle depth and evenness.

shading

Two or three shades of colour are applied to each 'slice' of hair. Semi-permanent colour can be used for a subtle look; tone-on-tone for visible colour; and permanent colour for a dramatic effect. This is a really good technique for thickening fine hair, as the multi-colour shading gives depth.

chunky lights

Normally applied on the top of the head and around the face, colour is added to wide-woven pieces of hair. Softer or stronger colours can be used to create different effects. This technique is best when slightly contrasting colours are used, as it will make the colour stand out.

bleaching

This technique is used to lighten hair or to create results that cannot be achieved with high-lift tint. Bleaching agents lighten the pigments of the hair and rinsing stops the process at the required shade. It's a job best left to the experts, as toning is a major part of this process.

duo/trio colour

A creative technique using tone-on-tone colour, which can be semi-permanent or permanent. Colour is applied in two sections to cover the whole head and can be subtle or dramatically different. Duo colour means two colours only; trio is three colours only.

waxes and pomades

Colour waxes or pomades are a totally temporary colouring method, ideal for those who like to go wild at the weekend but have to look smart during the week. It is applied after the hair has been dried and styled to give a dramatic look. If you have very blonde or bleached hair, do a test strand to make sure it doesn't stain the hair and will wash out.

tonal blast

The tips of the hair are first lightened and then tone-on-tone colour is applied. The lightened pieces of hair will show the tone more dramatically. This colour adds definition to shorter haircuts and works best when stronger colours, such as reds and coppers, are used.

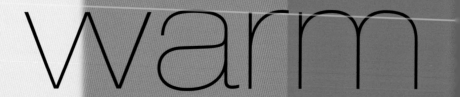

warm

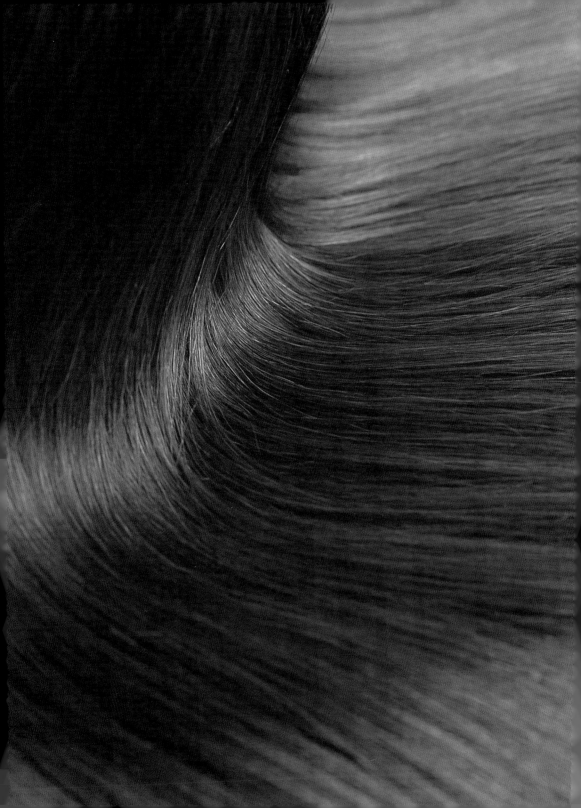

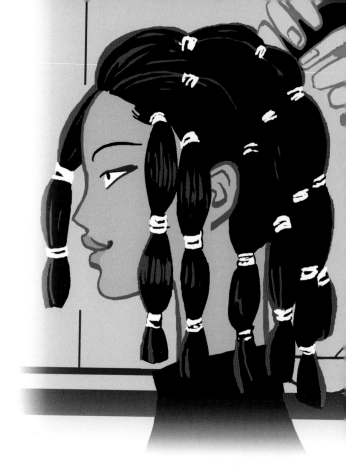

... jaz's creative-colour experience

Jaz's girlfriend, Vicci, whose passion for fashion equals Jaz's, has a younger sister who's a junior stylist at one of London's top salons. She's told them they're looking for models for creative colouring and, since Jaz has such great hair, would she be up for it? Stupid question! Jaz is there as quick as you can say highlights. She's been chosen for tie-dyeing – cool. What amazing timing with this party coming up at Shaft with Chrissie and the girls. She really wants to look hot – apparently it's going to be packed with movers and shakers from the media and the fashion pack. Jaz can hardly contain her excitement, which is not quite so cool, she realizes. While the hairstylist divides her hair into sections, she pictures herself working the room at Shaft and holding court, with a hip designer hanging on to her every word. These happy thoughts are interrupted by a serious style issue. What shade of nail polish will look best with her fuchsia-pink, bias-cut slip dress? Before she knows it (amazing how absorbing such matters can be), her hair has been sectioned with hair bands, scrunched up, coloured, washed and blow-dried. And – hey presto – her dark black, glossy locks are now mottled with variegated shades of red. Fab – it's just like the skirt she bought last weekend from Portobello market. Love it!

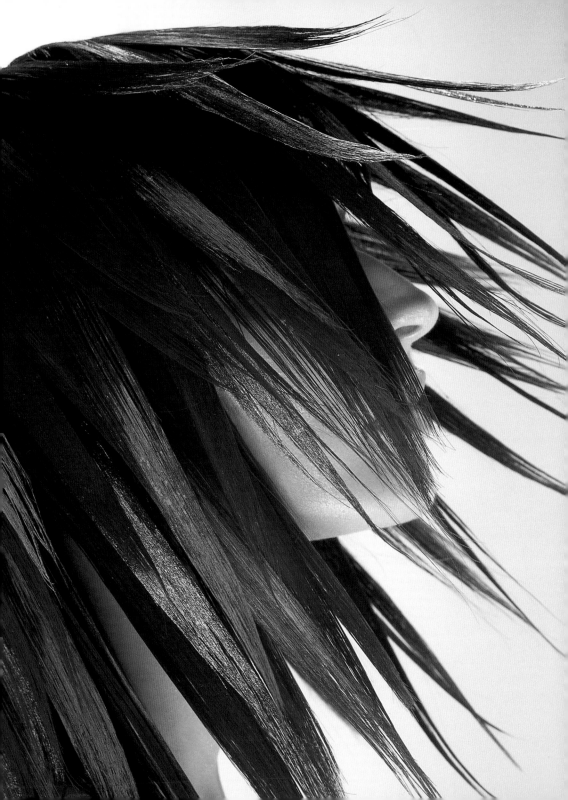

colouring tips

lighten up, but **not** at home

Attempting to lighten your hair yourself, using home-made preparations, lemon juice or – horror – bleach, is an extremely precarious business. Do without that must-have pair of feathered mules if need be, but leave your highlighting to the professionals. If you don't, you'll probably end up having to visit the salon anyway for a rescue job.

troubleshooting

If your hair has been coloured in a salon and you are unhappy with the end result, talk to your hairdresser; there are several things they can do. Colour can be masked or returned to your natural shade. Brassy or yellow bleached hair can be toned down with silvery or ashy temporary colour and a tint will also cover bleached hair. A colour stripper or reducer can also be used by your hairdresser to remove permanent tints. Repeated washing will lift semi-permanent colours, but this damages the condition of the hair, so always apply a protein-restructuring mask afterwards.

refresh your tresses

To revive your hair colour, use a colour enhancing shampoo and conditioner once a week. Always follow the manufacturer's instructions and leave them on for the specified time. Minuscule amounts of colour pigment will be deposited on the hair shaft to revitalize and maintain the colour. Vary this treatment with a shampoo and conditioner that has been specially formulated and designed to cope with the changes your hair has undergone.

shampoo/conditioner speak

Shampoos that have been specially formulated for colour-treated hair are designed to condition and cleanse the hair, as well as prevent the colour from fading. Conditioners formulated for colour-treated hair leave a protective film around porous, damaged areas of the hair shaft, helping to lock in the colour pigments and improve the condition of the hair, leaving it stronger and shinier.

don't be dull

If your hair has a tendency to look dull after it has been coloured, a good, quick and very natural treatment is to crack a raw egg onto your head after shampooing and work it through the hair. Leave it for five minutes and then rinse it out thoroughly. Top tip: Use cold or lukewarm water; if the water is too hot you will find that the egg will scramble and it will be difficult to remove. The natural proteins in eggs will leave the hair glossy and full of body.

natural remedy

If you find yourself in a fix without professional products, you can resort to Mother Nature. If your coloured hair has been in the sun and feels brittle and dry, mash up an avocado and work it into your hair after shampooing. Leave it on for at least five minutes to let the moisturizing oils penetrate the hair shaft, then rinse it off thoroughly.

fade out

If you find that your naturally brown hair starts to look dull and faded, steep three tea bags in a large jug of hot water, let it cool down and use it to rinse the hair. The natural dye in tea will even out and enhance the colour of your hair. Similarly, if your naturally blonde hair starts to look dull, rinse it with a solution of camomile tea made as described above. The antioxidant ingredients in the tea will leave your hair fresh, bright and glossy.

chlorine alert

Swimming in chlorinated water can turn bleached or blonde-tinted hair an unsightly shade of green. To prevent this, use products that have been specially designed to protect the hair in chlorinated water, and always rinse your hair immediately after swimming. To restore natural and enhanced blonde hair to its former glory, massage tomato juice into the hair after shampooing; leave for a few minutes and then rinse it out thoroughly. The active ingredients in the tomato juice will neutralize the green colour.

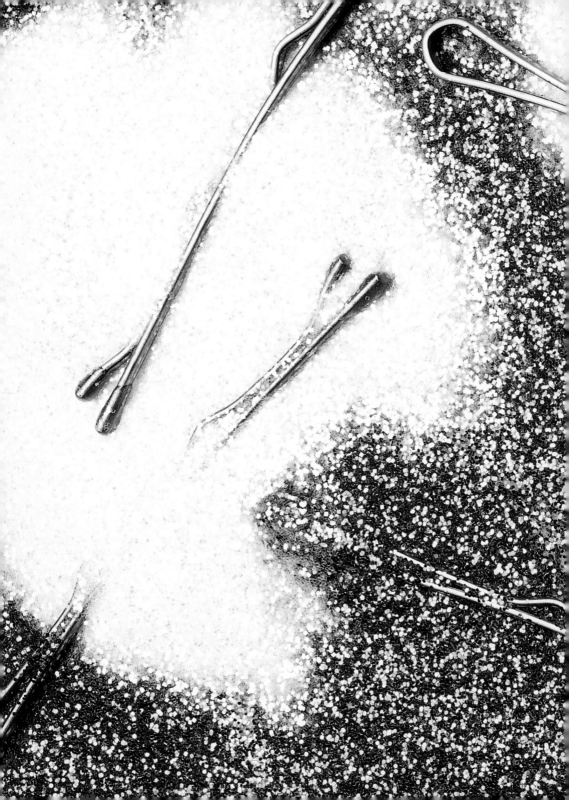

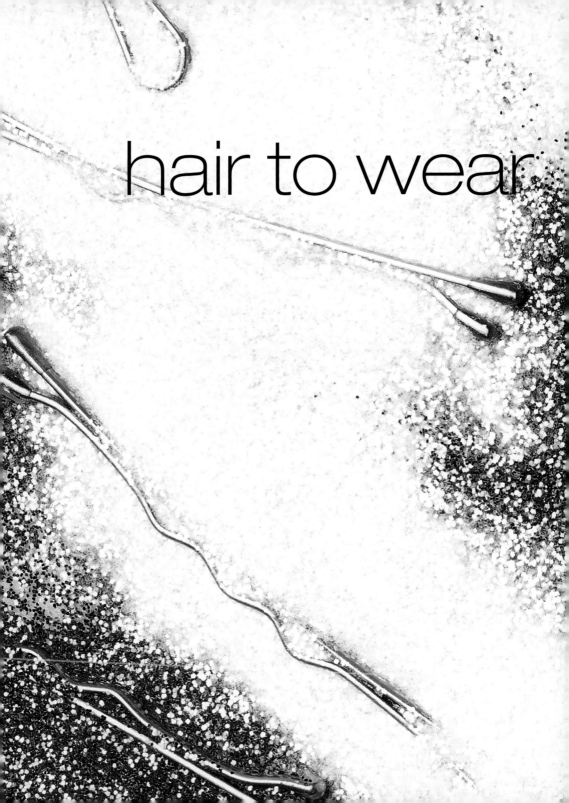
hair to wear

party prep at number 23

Saturday afternoon and very loud disco music was pumping out of the stereo over the non-stop whir of a hairdryer at number 23 Havana Road. There was definite excitement in the air. Chrissie was blow-drying Jaz's hair in the kitchen, Laura had just returned from her Fab Abs class at the gym and Polly was in her bedroom, packing for her trip to New York. In less than 12 hours, she would finally meet cyber-suitor Simon. His last e-mail had been especially flirtatious: 'Don't forget to bring your dancing shoes,' he had written. It usually took Polly 20 minutes tops to pack for a business trip, but today she had dithered for several hours and instead of her usual organized approach, clothes and shoes were strewn Chrissie-style across the bed. Dizzy with excitement, she finally tossed the scarlet camisole, a pair of high heels and a bias-cut slip dress into her case, along with the sensible navy business suits, of course. She jumped guiltily when Kate poked her head around the door to say goodbye, 'I'm off to the hairdressers. Have fun in New York, Pol.'

Kate was glad that she had a hair appointment to go to. Not only was the pounding music driving her mad, but the sight of their house guest running around in an endless selection of tight-fitting clothes – all flat stomach, long legs and sleek blonde hair – really was just too much. Still, it had increased Kate's resolve. After years of flowing, pre-Raphaelite locks and long floral dresses, the time had come to sharpen up her image and start climbing up that career ladder. She was even going to attend a Colour Me Beautiful session at a girlfriend's house that night. Matthew – her handsome boss, the marketing director – wouldn't recognize her on Monday.

At 6 pm Polly's cab arrived. 'Bye girls, I'm off now. Have a great time at the party,' she yelled above the music. Laura was trying to watch a political discussion on television while she waited for Jaz and Chrissie to make their grand entrances. She had been ready for hours, having showered and scrunched some mousse through her hair at the gym. She was pleased with her new, slightly wispier crop, although it'd seemed to have escaped the notice of the assistant producer in Current Affairs. She had no idea what this party would be like, but she'd pushed out the boat and had swapped her uniform of jeans and trainers for a slim-fitting skirt and – hell, it was worth a try – a spritz of 'Fatal'.

Jaz, meanwhile, had pulled out all the stops. She was desperate to wave goodbye to her job as a retail consultant at The Flag and land a plum position with a top designer. This party was the perfect opportunity for career enhancement, since it would be packed with fashionistas. Her new tie-dyed hair and matching red-and-black dip-dyed skirt ought to be enough to get her noticed.

Chrissie was also planning on having a little career advancement of her own. Determined to secure an audition – and a date – with Steve the producer, she had opted for 'result wear'.

Laura and Jaz gasped as she panthered into the living room. Her little black shell top was practically transparent, her heels as high as the Empire State Building and her fine, flyaway hair looked 'Big' with a capital 'B', thanks to some deft work with a hairdryer and styling product. 'Let's go, girls,' she cried.

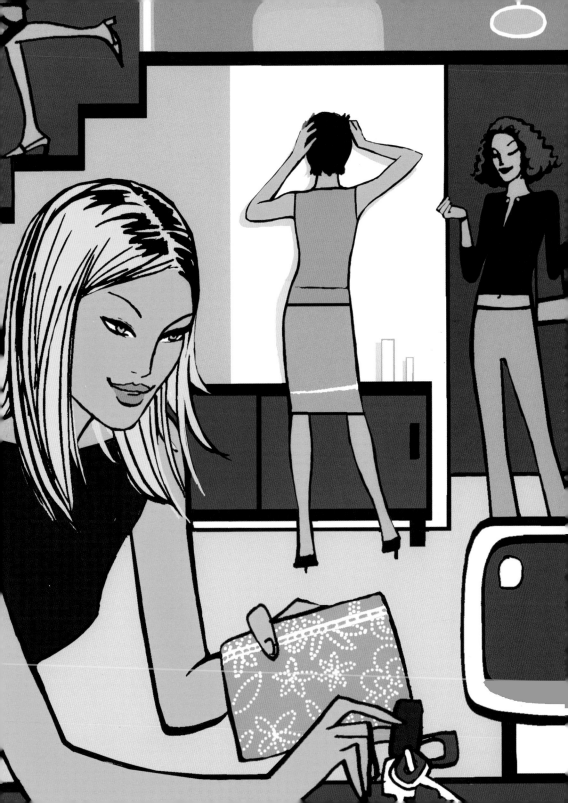

hair-styling

With a few good products and a little practice, anyone should be able to turn a bad-hair day into a good one. Learning how to use styling products effectively and achieving a good blow-dry at home are the first lessons. The critical point is the 'damp to dry' stage when hair has a style 'memory'. If you overdry your hair, spritz it with a little water from a plant mister.

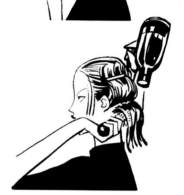

basic blow-dry

1 Gently pat as much moisture away from wet hair as possible using a towel. Rubbing the hair will ruffle the cuticles and causes tangles.

2 Hair loses one-quarter of its elasticity when it is wet, so gently comb it from the tips.

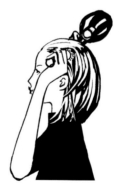

3 Tip your head upside-down and rough-dry your hair with the dryer on medium heat until it is 70 per cent dry. Lift and separate the hair at the roots and through the length with your fingers to create volume.

4 When the hair is still slightly damp, apply the styling product. Then section the back, top, fringe (bangs) and sides with big clips.

5 Starting at the back, unclip and style one section at a time. Use the brushes to lift the hair at the roots, then pull away to dry the length. Spend most effort and time on the front and side sections – once the frame to the face looks good, the rest follows.

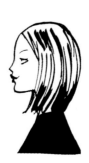

6 A fine shot of cool air on the hair, while still under brush control, will set the hair and close the cuticles, giving extra shine.

7 For the finishing touch, add a spot of serum for shine, a little wax to get a choppy look or just a spritz of hairspray to set the style.

HAIR SNIP

ALWAYS RUN THE HAIRDRYER DOWN THE LENGTH OF THE HAIR SHAFT TO KEEP THE CUTICLES LYING FLAT.

TIP YOUR HEAD UPSIDE-DOWN AND SPRAY HAIRSPRAY AT THE ROOTS FOR BIG VOLUME.

tool kit

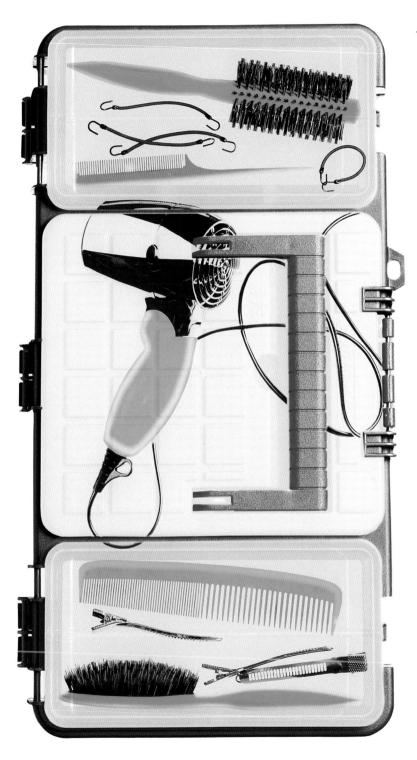

brushes

Your hairstyle will probably require at least two different brushes, depending on the hair length. One should be a round brush for smoothing or curling and the other a volumizing brush (see page 22).

hairdryer

Choose a hairdryer with a minimum strength of 1500 watts, several heat and force settings and a cold button for finishing.

products

Have to hand the appropriate mousse, gel, serum or styling spray for your particular type of hair and style (see page 21).

comb

A comb is used for, careful detangling, sectioning off hair for styling and for creating partings.

clips

These hold sections of hair out of the way while you are blow-drying and styling.

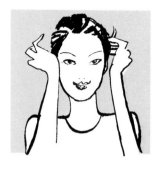

natural drying

1 Start by evenly applying your chosen styling product using your fingers and finishing with a comb.

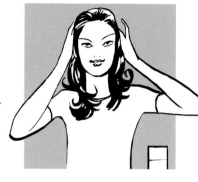

2 'Mould' your hair into the desired shape before drying it to ensure a perfect finish.

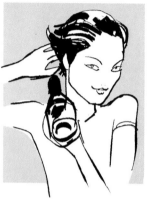

3 Start drying your hair, using your fingers as a brush. This will give maximum lift at the roots.

4 Dry all sections thoroughly and then finish using a light wax.

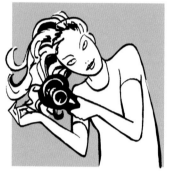

great curls

1 Apply a styling product that is suitable for your hair type – it is really important to start with a great foundation.

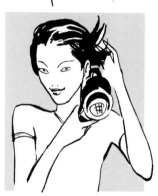

2 Tip your head to one side and, using the bowl of the diffuser, lift the hairdryer up and down into the hair with a gentle movement. Then tip your head to the other side and repeat.

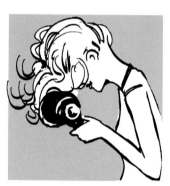

3 When the hair is dry, tip your head forward and carry on with a similar motion. If you find your hair is starting to go fluffy, spritz it with a shine spray.

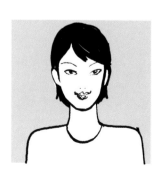

4 When you have finished all the sections of the hair, gently run a serum evenly through it to create a more defined curl.

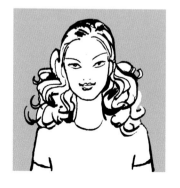

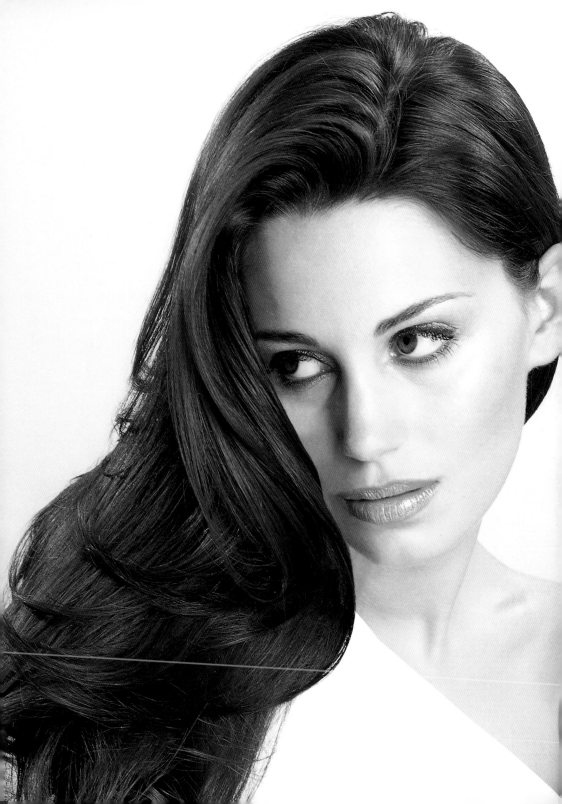

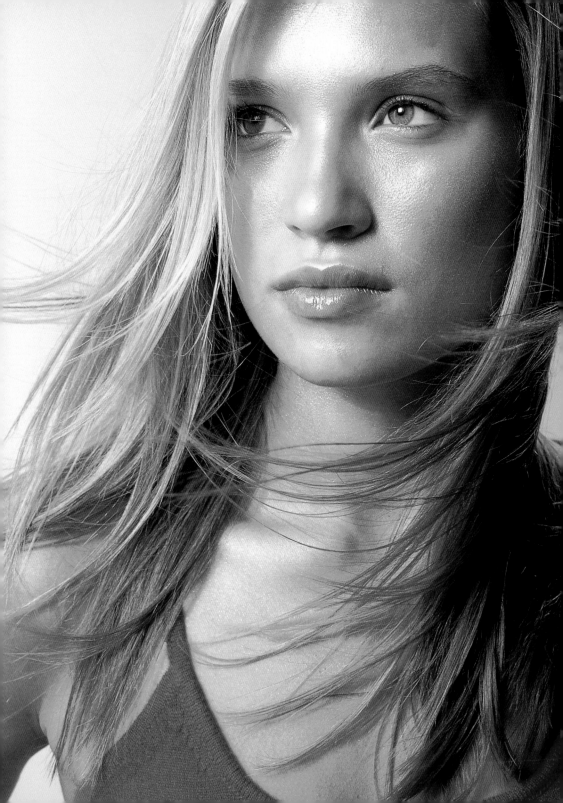

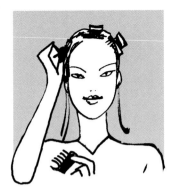

straightening

Here are some step-by-step tips for taming your tresses to create bone-straight sleek hair.

1 Start by applying your chosen product evenly through the hair – an anti-frizz serum is ideal.

2 Beginning at the back, use clips to section the hair. Avoid taking too big a section.

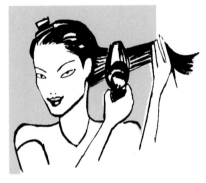

3 Using a paddle brush, dry each section in a downwards motion. Start at the roots, taking the brush right through to the ends of the hair. To finish each section, give the hair a blast of cold air.

4 When all the sections of the hair are dry, lightly spray with hairspray to seal the cuticles.

5 Heat the straightening irons and, when they are very hot, run them from the roots to the ends of the hair to ensure Cleopatra-style straight hair. This will seal the cuticles of the hair, leaving it almost impossible for any moisture to penetrate the shaft.

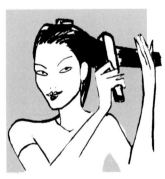

6 To complete the look, spray the hair with a light mist of glossing spray.

HAIR SNIP

IF THERE IS A LOT OF MOISTURE IN THE AIR, OR IT IS VERY HUMID, USE AN ANTI-HUMIDITY SPRAY. THESE CONTAIN ANTI-HUMECTANTS WHICH SEAL THE HAIR AND BLOCK MOISTURE. A LEAVE-IN CONDITIONER WILL ALSO HELP PREVENT YOUR SLEEK LOCKS FROM BECOMING A FRIZZY MESS. ALTERNATIVELY, MIX TWO PARTS OF GEL WITH ONE PART OF SERUM AND APPLY IT TO WET HAIR.

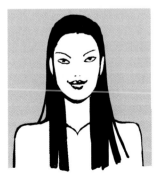

quick fixes

1 If your hair is short, try slicking it back into a sleek crop or simply use pretty pins to decorate it.

2 If your hair is dirty, pin it up. Day-old hair is always easier to put up and will stay in place better than freshly washed hair. Turn unclean hair to your advantage by making a finger-combed ponytail on the crown of your head (avoid too much brushing as this increases the oiliness) and tie it with an elastic. Twist a length of hair around the elastic, fixing it with grips as you go. Let locks of different lengths twist out if they want to; the more effortless the look, the higher the glam factor.

3 If your hair is curly, revitalize it by spritzing it with water and gently scrunching. If it has become frizzy, work a little serum through each tendril, tackling it section by section.

4 If your hair is flat, try a little backcombing to give it lift. Start at the crown and work your way around to the sides. You don't need to backcomb all over, just enough to give a little lift.

5 Do not try to slick back dirty hair with copious amounts of wet-look gel. Although it looks good in magazines, in reality no one is fooled.

6 Never underestimate how long it takes to wash and dry your hair. Forfeit a shampoo for a spot of inventive yet speedy styling.

7 If you are not confident with grips and combs (quick-fix 1), it is better to shower and leave with fresh, clean-smelling but perhaps damp hair than to get frustrated in front of a mirror.

8 Keep an emergency hair kit in the car or office that includes: a brush, a cordless straightener or curling iron, the nearly finished bottles of mousse and serum from home, and a few grips and elastics that can save the day.

9 When you get given another hairdryer for Christmas, take one to the office. It is amazing how many times you get caught in the rain.

10 If your hair is really greasy and you have no time to wash it, apply some dry shampoo or talc close to the roots. Massage it in gently to absorb the excess oil and then brush it out. Or, use cotton wool to dab a little witch hazel onto the roots to absorb any grease.

style-and-go tips

1 To control static, flyaway hair, simply spray a comb with hairspray and gently run it through your locks.

2 Cheap shampoos containing strong detergents will strip your hair of its natural oils and make it seem dull, lank and lifeless.

3 If your hair is very tangled, work it through with a comb first before you begin to use your brush. This will cause as little damage as possible.

4 Keep it cool. Using a hairdryer on a cool setting is good for the scalp, especially if you have greasy hair. Apply too much heat and the scalp will perspire for up to 15 minutes after you've finished drying, causing your hair to drop and lose its shape. It will also activate the oil-producing glands. Whatever your hair type, avoid overdrying, too.

5 Sleep on a satin pillowcase to avoid 'bed-head' hair. In the night your hair will slide gently across it, whereas cotton causes friction which can disrupt the hair cuticles.

6 If, on the other hand, you want to acheive 'bed-head' hair, apply mousse to slightly damp hair before you go to bed. In the morning, simply arrange into place with styling wax or pomade.

7 To keep the hair shaft blunt and prevent split ends, have a trim at least every six weeks.

8 Touch your hair as little as possible after styling it. Otherwise it will lose its shape and body and could become greasy.

9 Simple styles can be energized with temporary colour. Try using hair mascara in bright blue or black for an extra-daring look.

10 To reduce the effects of static hair in the mornings, wrap your hair loosely in a silk headscarf before going to bed. (Probably only worth trying if you sleep alone!)

11 To avoid flat hair, make sure your hair is totally dry when you go to bed. With slightly damp hair, you may well wake up with a frizzy mop, and it's more likely to be flat against your scalp.

12 Two-in-one products can be a great timesaver, but avoid using those that are silicone-based. These build up a coating on the hair which makes it difficult to style.

interview hair

Big hair with lots of root lift was where stylish hair was at in the 1980s – think of the stars of *Dynasty* and *Dallas*. Thankfully, though, these days hair that means business is definitely sleek, easy and under control. The thinking being that if you can't keep your hair under control, how can you possibly be keeping your business under control either? Groomed hair is smart-and-together hair; a sleek ponytail, a smart, short crop or a bob are the perfect styles, and shiny, silky hair in tip-top condition is a must.

It is often quoted that employers decide in the first three minutes into an interview who they are going to employ. To make a good impression, ensure your hair is clean and shiny, as it is an obvious sign that you take care of yourself – the thinking being that if you don't take care of yourself, will you take care of your job? Make sure that your hair is not overly elaborate. If a style looks like it takes an age to create, you will be sending out signals that you will be wasting company time checking your reflection in mirrors. Leave elaborate hairstyles to ladies who lunch, who have nothing more important on their minds than their next Caesar salad. A ponytail can be elegant, but girly styles like plaits and braiding are a no-no if you want to be taken seriously. Depending on the type of business, leave the pink bow and glitter hair slides for the evening. Your Hello Kitty hair accessories won't impress a bank or law firm.

2 Your hairdresser can show you how to attach a hairpiece in the same colour as your own hair to add bulk to a thin ponytail.

3 Avoid tying your hair back towards the crown. Positioned too high, your chic updo will become a cheerleader's ponytail.

4 Keep a hairpiece for ponytails handy on business trips. That way, even if you don't have time to wash your hair, you can tie it back, slick it down and look super-stylish in a moment.

5 Wrap a small strand of hair around the elastic so that it can't be seen and fix it with a grip on the underside. It finishes off the look better than a hair accessory. Alternatively, to make sure your ponytail is really secure, use wet string instead of an elastic to hold it. The string will contract as it dries, fixing the hair in place. As before, wrap a small section of hair around the string to hide it.

6 Slick down wispy bits with a little serum and hairspray to keep the look sleek rather than sporty.

7 If your hair is fine and flyaway, wash it the day before so it's easier to handle and stays in place.

updos

Sleek, chic and giving the appearance of being effortlessly elegant and well-groomed, long hair pinned up in a chignon always means business. Even simpler ponytails can work just as well on hair that is layered or growing out as on straight, one-length hair.

1 Tidy up growing-out layers and feather-cuts by combing through some holding mousse before tying back the hair.

power bobs

The simple bob – with or without a fringe (bangs); curled-up, curled-under or straight; short or long; blunt-cut or wispy – always means business. There is a variation to suit everyone, so talk to your hairdresser about finding the one that suits you. It can be made sleeker or choppier with styling products, depending on your mood. It is the versatility of the bob that keeps it so fresh, even though it has been around since the 1920s.

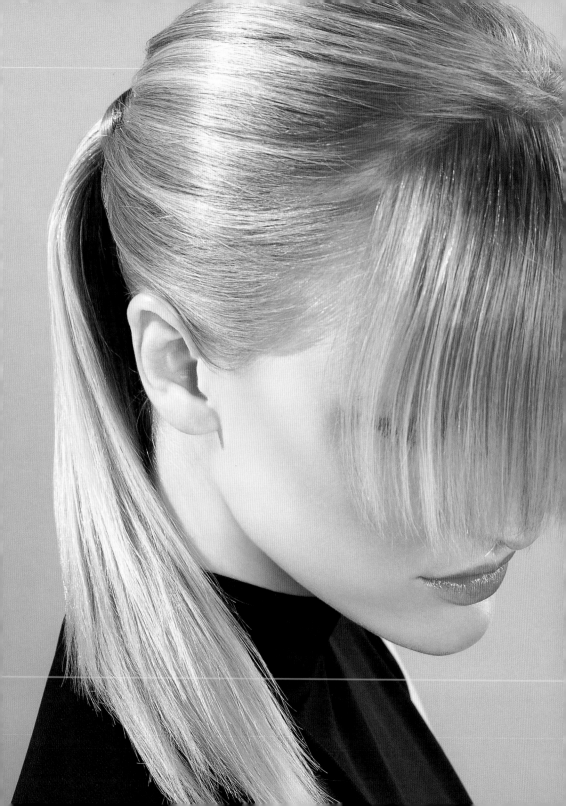

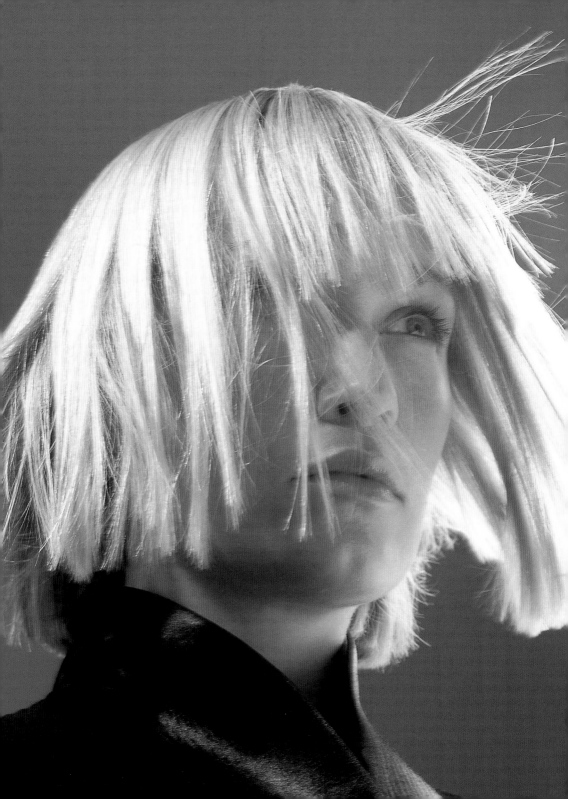

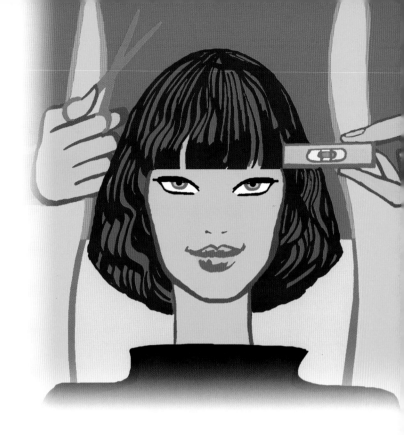

... kate's take on a power bob

Kate can't bear the thought of looking like a cross between a 1970s throwback from the easy-care perm days and Goldilocks for one minute longer. With her crush on Matthew the marketing director growing more intense by the week, Kate is increasingly interested in how she appears at work. While munching her way through a packet of the latest Crunch biscuits (all in the name of research), she'd read a magazine article entitled confidently 'How to Get Ahead at Work'. Point number three, which was all about image and self-

projection, had made quite an impression. With new resolve – a woman with a mission – she hurtles to the hairdresser and demands a power bob (also advised in the very same article). Her patient stylist explains that a classic power bob is a no-no with her hair type; it was never going to look like Uma Thurman's poker-straight 'do' in *Pulp Fiction*. What he can do, though, is a give her a sleeker, more groomed look, by taking off some length, adding some layers and generally tidying up her tresses into a bob shape.

Kate starts feeling calmer and her breathing becomes more regulated as she watches herself being transformed into Miss Get Ahead at Work (and, more to the point, Miss How to Get Mr Marketing Director to Look Twice). Her stylist suggests blow-drying her hair straight (the closest she will ever get to a true power bob). Kate can't believe her eyes – she looks like Julia Roberts with sleek hair at the Oscars (sort of). Mr MD – wake up and smell the coffee! For the first time in her life, Kate can't wait to get to work on Monday.

work to play

The invite is for drinks at 7:30, or dinner at 8, yet you know you won't finish work until 6:30 at the earliest. Even if you do get off early, there is no way you can negotiate the cross-town, rush-hour traffic, get changed and get back in time. If you try (and everyone has done it once), you end up frazzled, in a foul temper and 30 minutes late. How much better, then, to make the work-to-play transition in the office or at a nearby gym.

One advantage of choosing a hairstylist near your office is that many salons now offer beauty treatments and have showering facilities available. Build a good relationship with your stylist and you will never have to change at work again. If an invite is sprung on you at the last moment and you have no change of clothes, it is amazing how a professional blow-dry can improve your spirits and your appearance. Your boring suit and white T-shirt suddenly look pared-down and Calvin Klein-ish with an expert coiff. If the salon option is out of the question, opt for one of these styles or try one of the quick fixes on page 62.

twisted sister

1 Start by dividing all of the hair into 5-cm (2-in) square sections. Use sectioning clips to hold them out of the way.

2 Starting at the nape, take each section individually and twist it tightly from the root through to the ends. As you work your way up each section, you'll find that it starts to twist down onto itself. Let this happen until it is sitting on your starting point, then secure it in place with a matt grip.

3 Repeat this, working your way up the head to the crown, until you have twisted each section.

4 Finish by spritzing with a non-aerosol hairspray, which will ensure a strong hold.

glam-hair updo

1 Loosely tie your hair back in a ponytail using a snag-free elastic to maintain a strong hold.

2 Lightly backcomb the ponytail section to create extra volume.

3 Fold sections of the ponytail into the middle of the head, securing them in place with matt grips placed close to the elastic. This can be random – the beauty of the style is that it should look as if you've done it yourself.

4 When all of the hair is secured, lightly apply non-aerosol hairspray.

5 Choose an accessory to suit your outfit.

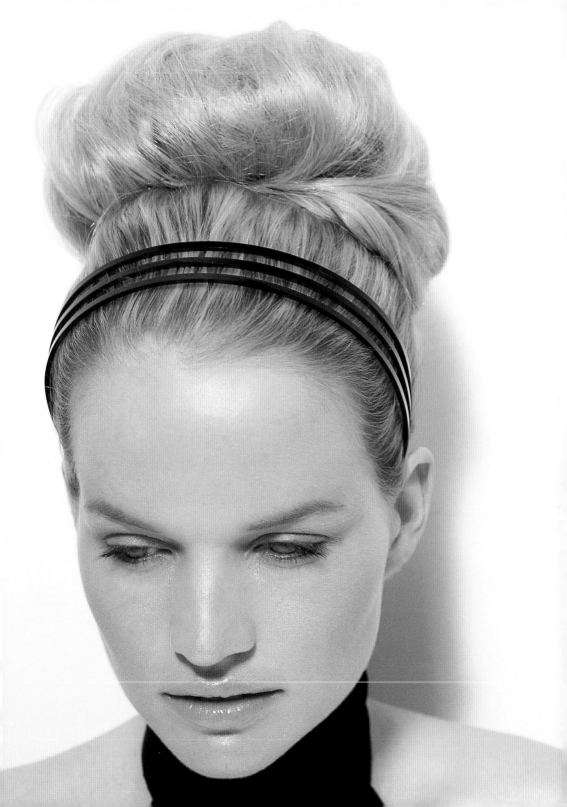

jet-set hair

Relatively inexpensive air travel has given most of us fast access to the 'global village'. Air travel was once strictly for the jet set, but now that it is no longer exclusive, no one pretends (not even the first-class passengers) that they feel glamorous after a 14-hour flight. Even though the wellbeing programmes on in-flight entertainment give tips on how to exercise (isn't sitting with your knees under your chin exercise?) and avoid dehydration, they never mention how to keep your hair looking as good on arrival as it did on departure.

dehydration

The air pressure in the cabin and the high altitude encourage dehydration, which leaves the skin and hair dull and lacking in radiance. This can only be prevented by drinking copious amounts of water and soft drinks, while avoiding tea, coffee and alcohol, all of which have a diuretic effect that will compound the problem. Drinking carrot and apple juice before a flight will also help to keep hair hydrated.

static

The dry, air-conditioned cabin atmosphere could not be better for static, nor worse for flyaway hair (the wispy rather than the jet-set sort). If you have ever tried brushing or combing your hair while sitting in your seat, you will know that you can hear the crackle of static over the noise of the engines. While there is nothing you can do to change the climate in the cabin, you can counter the static by fixing hair in place with holding wax and gels, which give the hair weight. Resting a headscarf over the headrest will also help to reduce the friction between your hair and the back of the seat.

flaky scalp

Dehydration on board means an increased chance of developing a flaky scalp. If this has happened to you, tie back your hair to avoid dandruff-like flakes on your shoulders. Once you are settled in at your destination, a vigorous but gentle brushing will loosen any flakes.

Follow with a thorough scalp massage to increase the blood flow, and therefore nutrients and oxygen, to the scalp, as well as to release tension from the flight (see page 24). Finally, a shampoo and deep-conditioning treatment will remove any lingering flakes and restore moisture, bounce and shine.

Air-hair dos and don'ts

Don't fly with your hair weighted down with products or your face caked with panstick. Fly with clean hair and a slick of lipstick, if you like.

Do spritz your face regularly with a hydrating mister to keep the skin soft and supple. Use it to refresh stale, dry hair, too.

Do drink plenty of still mineral water.

Don't drink coffee, tea or alcohol.

Do always pack your skincare and haircare products in waterproof bags so there's no chance of them spilling their contents over your favourite silk dress.

Do tie your hair back to help prevent static building up. If you do get static hair, spray some hairspray onto your brush or comb and lightly run it through the hair.

Do pack a gentle, restorative shampoo and super-rich conditioner to revive your travel-stressed hair on arrival.

Do not despair. If you still look less-than-perfect on arrival – despite the litres of water and a first-class seat – simply act like a filmstar and don a pair of dark 'Jackie O' sunglasses, a smart hat, a slick of red lipstick and a disenchanted air.

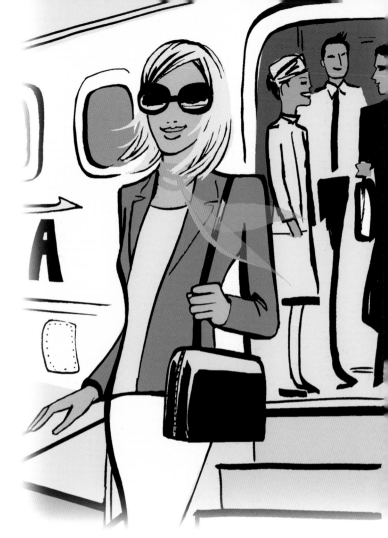

Never before has the prospect of a business trip to New York seemed quite so exciting as it does now. Apart from the obvious retail opportunities, it's the anticipation of finally meeting cyber-suitor Simon, who has her heart fluttering like a teenager's. There is one problem, though – aeroplane hair – and she has to go straight out from JFK to a dinner meeting uptown with no time for a hotel stop and hair overhaul. After a few hours of being subjected to the two demon hair enemies – static and

... polly's air-hair dilemma

dehydration – Polly's worried that she'll disembark with hair so frizzy and static that the only spark between her and Simon will be the electric shock she gives him when they shake hands for the first time. What to do? Hair in bun? Business-like but maybe too prim. Wear a headscarf? Ladylike-chic but a bit too HRH.

A baseball cap? Very American but not a good look with a suit. Polly hits a brick wall, but a quick phone call to her hair guru, Charles, solves the problem. Drink plenty of H_2O and – top tip – a carrot and apple juice before flying to combat dehydration. Another top tip, put a headscarf on the headrest to prevent static

from the nylon seat covers. Hah! She knew the headscarf would come in handy. Armed with bottles of water and various fruit juice concoctions, her Hermès scarf knotted around her neck, Polly sashays down the corridors at Heathrow's Terminal 4 without a second thought for her boyfriend. Sorry, Harry.

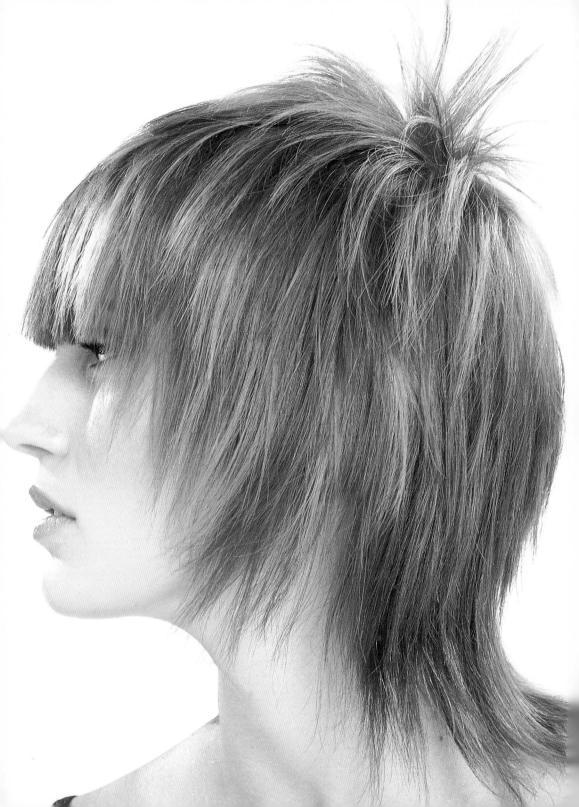

vive la change

We all know someone who has taken the plunge and had the big chop. It usually coincides with a big life change, invariably the end of a relationship. Cutting long hair short is a liberation and, when one considers how men prize long hair, it is a form of emancipation from their – his – ideals. There is bravery attached to a dramatic new look, too. A complete change of colour or a cut – or both – can be tremendously energizing and rejuvenating. Some people thrive on change, whereas others need a gentle nudge to pluck up the courage.

considerations

Whether you're the sort of person who gets a real buzz from reinventing yourself or you take the cautious approach, don't do anything rash. Think carefully about your new look, consider all the options and ask advice from your stylist. The decision to chop off a good four years' growth of hair should not be taken lightly.

1 Think about why you want to have a dramatic change. Remember, a haircut won't bring a lover back or put the world to rights, but it might restore your confidence, perk up your mood and give you a much-needed boost.

2 Are you prepared to change your wardrobe and make-up to accommodate a dramatic new hairstyle? For example, if you are naturally a long-haired brunette, having a short blonde crop will affect the colouring of your face and different clothes will suit you. Be prepared.

3 Copying someone else's style to the letter never works successfully. Find a style or cut that inspires you, then, with the help of your hairstylist, make it your own.

4 A flexible hairstyle is the best one to have. You may love your spiky crop when it's just been done, but get bored with it after the initial impact has worn off.

5 Colour, rather than cut, is the easiest way to effect a big change and yet still leave you with the option to reverse it. A cut is more permanent as it grows out slowly, at little more than 1 cm (½ in) a month.

6 If you are considering cutting long hair, try on a few short-styled wigs beforehand to make sure you like the way it looks on you.

7 If you are thinking of growing out a short haircut, use hairpieces to see if you like the feel of longer hair.

8 Make sure you're ready for a change and don't let anyone push you into doing anything you're not happy about.

9 Think of the upkeep. Will your new look be easy or an effort to style? Will it fit in with your lifestyle? How versatile do you need it to be? And how often will you need to revisit the hairdresser to keep it looking good?

HAIR SNIP

WHEN YOU'RE CONSIDERING GOING FOR A COMPLETE IMAGE-OVERHAUL, LOOK THROUGH LOTS OF BEAUTY AND FASHION MAGAZINES TO FIND AS MANY PICTURES AS YOU CAN OF HAIRSTYLES AND HAIR COLOURS THAT YOU LIKE. TAKE THE WHOLE SELECTION WITH YOU TO THE HAIRDRESSER'S AND YOUR STYLIST WILL HELP YOU DECIDE WHAT ELEMENTS FROM EACH LOOK WILL SUIT YOU AND YOUR HAIR TYPE. THAT WAY, YOU CAN CREATE A UNIQUE LOOK.

gently does it

If you like the idea of changing your image but just can't seem to pluck up the courage to go for a complete reinvention, try a few subtle, temporary changes first. Ask your hairstylist to blow-dry your hair in a different way – if you are naturally curly, get them to blow-dry it dead straight; if you normally wear it forwards, framing your face, ask them to style it away from your face; or have it set in curlers to create gentle waves. If you always wear your hair loose, ask your hairdresser to show you a new way of pinning it up; or simply try parting it in a different way. You could even have a semi-permanent colour rinse that will wash out in a few weeks. All of these devices can make you look and feel quite different without committing yourself to a radical change that will take years to reverse.

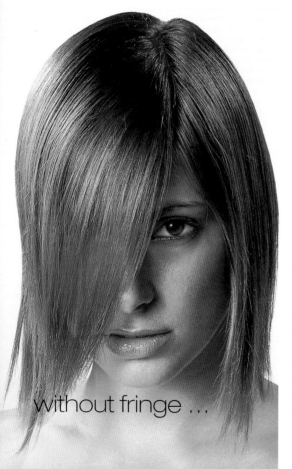

without fringe ...

If you are flirting with the idea of having short hair, then think about moving up in stages rather than going for a crop in one fell swoop of the scissors. You could evolve from a one-length long cut to a layered Rachel cut, then a shoulder-length bob or a sexy layered 'rock chick' style. You can then try a messed-up Meg Ryan cut and still have hair left to go even shorter. Gradual change is experimental and will give you time to play ideas out and find which styles and cuts suit your face and your personality most.

to fringe or not to fringe?

There are no hard and fast rules about hair type or face shape: some people simply do not suit fringes (bangs). It's a very personal thing. If you are thinking of having a fringe but are not sure if it will suit you, or if you fancy a fringe but don't want anything permanent which you will then have to grow out (a big bore), try faking it. It sounds unlikely but it does work!

How to do it: take a section of hair from the crown, comb it forwards over your forehead and arrange it as you would a fringe. If you've got long hair, twist it to take away the length before taking it forwards. Adjust the width, length and density as required, then clip it securely just above the crown using a large grip. Alternatively, ask your hairstylist to attach a hairpiece. Leave your false fringe for 20 minutes to get used to it before deciding whether it suits you.

moving on

Even the most dramatic changes lose their impact after a time, so the trick is to reinvent your look to avoid getting stuck in a style rut. Think how differently Madonna looks at 40 compared with how she looked in her twenties. Many feel she looks younger now. True to type, she has grown her hair and left it long at the age when most women feel they have to go short. Luckily, hair does grow. So unlike that dolphin tattoo swimming across your buttock, even the most radical change of colour and cut will grow out over time. Be brave and enjoy the positive power of transformation that a radical change can bring. (See overleaf – would you do it?)

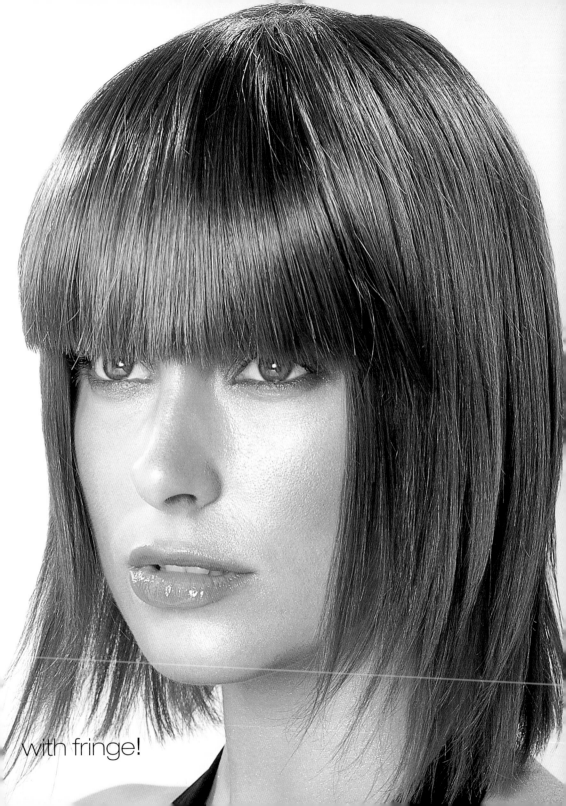

with fringe!

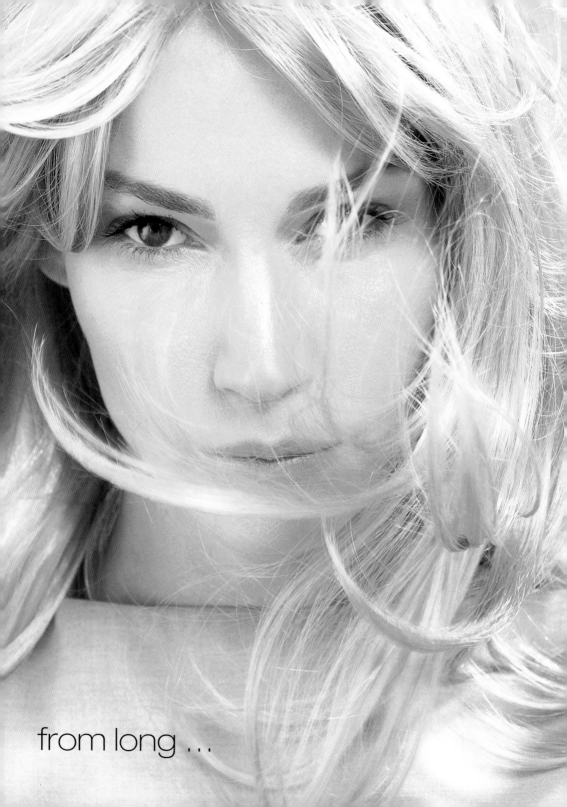

from long …

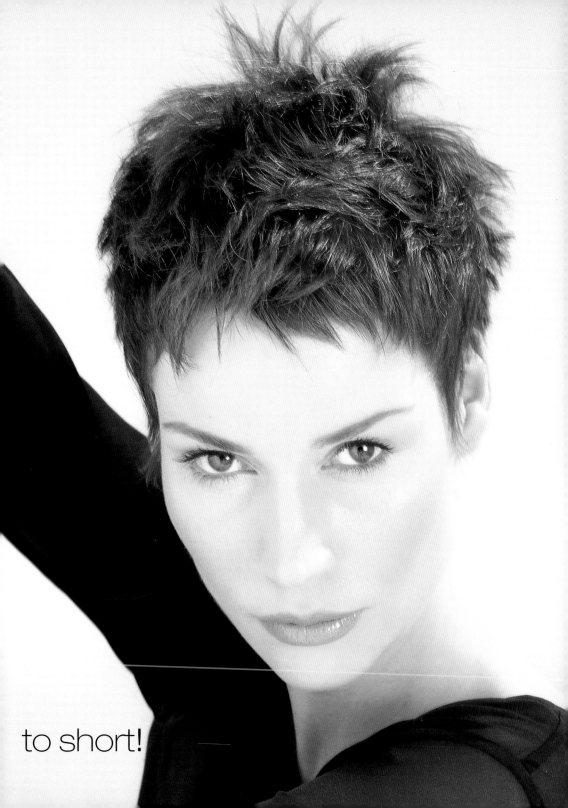

to short!

disco divas party on

Jaz simply could not believe her luck. Squashed up at the bar of Shaft with Laura, while attempting to order yet another round of Cosmopolitans, she'd struck up a conversation with a girl called Imogen, who turned out to be … wait for it … the fashion editor on *Gloss* magazine.

'Sweetie, I love your two-tone hair,' Imogen had declared to Jaz by way of a conversation opener. Jaz, in return, had admired Imogen's fluorescent pink mules, and before she knew it she'd been offered an (unpaid) work placement on *Gloss*. Jaz didn't think twice about accepting. She would quit her job at The Flag on Monday, even if it meant taking an evening job to pay the rent.

In another corner of the crowded bar, Chrissie had Steve the record producer well and truly under her spell – or so she thought. She had been flirting with him relentlessly all evening, purring into his ear and batting her eyelids until she was dizzy. 'Honey, this is a fabulous party … so glad we were able to come along … there are always so many invitations on Saturday nights.' Laura and Jaz listened in to snatches of the conversation, most impressed by Chrissie's small talk, if not by her taste in men.

'OK, Chrissie,' Steve was saying. 'Here's the deal. I'll arrange the interview with Pout. But there's something I want to ask you in return.'
'Yes, honey?' Chrissie flashed him her most winning smile. The audition was in the bag; now he was going to ask her out on a date.
'I was wondering if we could go out to dinner. Sort of a double date – you, me, your flatmate and a friend of mine, John. You see, I really like … Laura.'
Laura! Chrissie practically fell off her skyscraper heels, but thought quickly. Not only was it in the interests of her pop career to go on a double date with Steve, but over three courses and a few bottles of wine she knew she could convince him that it was she, Chrissie, in whom he should be interested. Not boyish, trainer-wearing Laura.
'Oh, I'm sure I can fix up something,' Chrissie purred through gritted teeth.

'No way,' whispered Laura to Jaz. 'He wears leather pants and he looks like a creep. I'm not going on a date with him.' But she hadn't factored in Chrissie's powers of persuasion. By the time the girls left Shaft at 3 am the audition, the double date and a job on *Gloss* were all secured. Result all round – if not exactly what Chrissie had planned.

Across town, poor Kate was swallowing the truly disastrous news that her colour palette should be oyster pinks, peach and … biscuit. Yep, apparently she had to dress in the same shade as a stale digestive in order to get herself noticed at Crunch Biscuits. Life was so unfair; no doubt Prissie Chrissie would be a strawberry-cream or a chocolate-coated cookie.

Meanwhile, on the other side of the pond, Polly's plane was about to touch down at JFK. She hadn't had a wink of sleep – too many glasses of water and trips to the ghastly loos. And she'd also been too busy feeling guilty about Harry and wondering if cyber-suitor Simon was as sexy as he sounded in his e-mails. Very soon, she would find out.

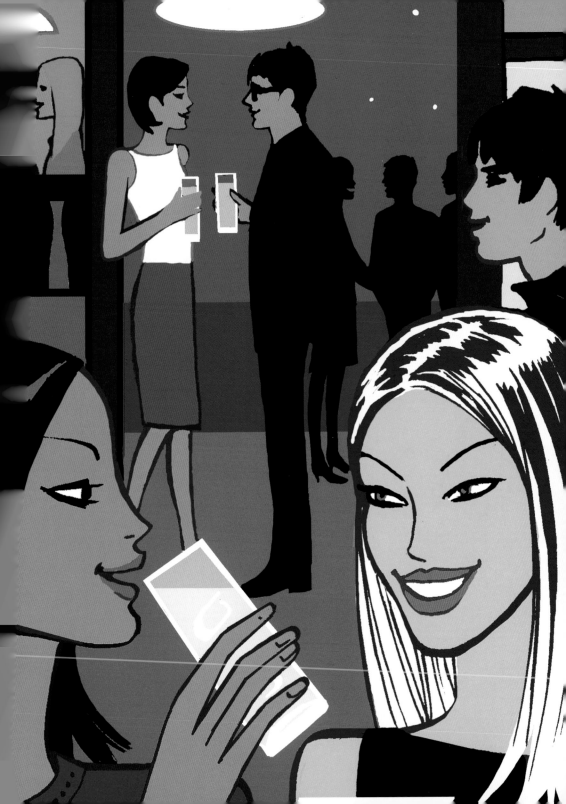

acknowledgements

Thank you to Adam Reed and Carolyn Newman at the
Percy Street salon. With special thanks to
Julie Gibson Jarvie, Penny Stock and Venetia Penfold,
without whom the book wouldn't have been possible.

The publishers would like to thank Joseph (020 7225 3335)
and Amanda Wakeley (0207 590 9105)
for fashion loans for the shoot.